the
Hepatitis C
cookbook

easy and delicious recipes

Heather Jeanne

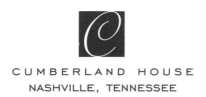

CUMBERLAND HOUSE
NASHVILLE, TENNESSEE

Published by
Cumberland House Publishing
431 Harding Industrial Drive
Nashville, Tennessee 37211

Cover design: Unlikely Suburban Design
Text design: Mary Sanford

Library of Congress Cataloging-in-Publication Data
Jeanne, Heather, 1970-
   The hepatitis C cookbook : easy and delicious recipes / Heather Jeanne ; foreword by Kev Krueger ; introduction by Eugene Somner.
        p. cm.
   Includes index.
   ISBN 1-58182-418-1 (pbk. : alk. paper)
   1. Hepatitis C—Diet therapy—Recipes. I. Title.
   RC848.H425J43 2004
   616.3'6230654--dc22
                                                              2004018741

Printed in Canada
1 2 3 4 5 6 7—10 09 08 07 06 05 04

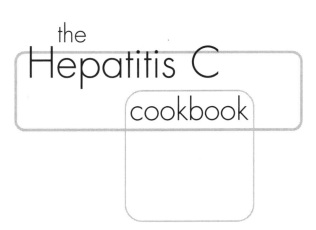

the
Hepatitis C
cookbook

Dedicated to my father, Franklin DeLano, one of the many thousands of hepatitis C sufferers; Beverly Schulz, whose teaching inspired me to continue to dream; the Fiorino family; Andy and Wanda Burt; Mom and Dad Maybury, whose support has been priceless; Mom and Dad, for loving and accepting me for who I am; and Melanie Maybury Huetter, my best friend.

contents

foreword

Hepatitis C is a potentially fatal virus that attacks the liver. According to the Centers for Disease Control, between eight and ten thousand Americans die each year from the disease, and it is now the leading cause of liver transplantation. Hepatitis C has already infected an estimated four to five million Americans and its worldwide impact may be as high as 200 million victims. Most experts agree that if the rate of hepatitis C infection isn't curbed soon, it will eventually kill more people each year than AIDS.

Early diagnosis continues to be a problem with hepatitis C because its victims don't normally develop symptoms until ten to twenty years after initial infection. Symptoms can vary significantly from person to person and may include fatigue, nausea, abdominal pain, irritability, depression, pain in the area of the liver, headaches, loss of appetite, dark urine, foggy-headedness, jaundice, and malaise.

Unfortunately, by the time symptoms appear, many will already have sustained liver damage that may become life-threatening. The good news is that many patients never develop symptoms, and the medical establishment believes that only 30 percent of those infected will see their disease progress to cirrhosis and/or liver cancer. The majority of folks with hepatitis C will likely continue living normal lives except for the knowledge that they are living with a contagious virus. Even so, it's a good idea for anyone who's been infected with this virus to follow a wellness program that emphasizes nutrition and healthy living.

There is no cure for hepatitis C, but it can most definitely be controlled. Three of the most important areas that patients need to think about are:

1. Protecting the liver from ongoing damage.
2. Boosting immunity, which the virus is known to suppress in humans.
3. Keeping the liver detoxified.

All of the above can be accomplished by numerous methods, but patients need to be mindful of their importance because they can literally make the difference in whether or not the disease becomes life-threatening.

It's no secret that those who take an active role in their own health usually fare much better through illness than those who rely solely on their doctors to "fix" them. I believe this is especially true for those of us who are infected with hepatitis C. Of all the lifestyle changes we can make to help ourselves heal and feel better, eating healthy meals is probably one of the easiest and most beneficial. The right foods can not only help alleviate symptoms, but they can also help us fight the disease!

To heal and function at its best, the liver must receive the many nutrients it needs. Most doctors recommend that hepatitis C patients eat small meals throughout the day to do this, rather than eating the usual "big three" that most of us are accustomed to. This prevents the liver from having to work so hard and feeds the liver nutrients continuously throughout the day. Unfortunately though, it isn't always so easy for those like myself who have problems with appetite caused by the disease. I force myself to eat because I know I need to and feel better when I do, but this just further underscores the need to prepare meals that are not only pleasing to the eye and tasty to the palate, but nutritious and healing to the liver as well. This book will teach you how to do this and more!

I was diagnosed with hepatitis C in 1994. I learned early on how important diet would be to my continued health. In spite of all the challenges, I've found that a hepatitis C diagnosis doesn't have to mean the end of joy and pleasure. Happiness, even with hepatitis C, is a choice, plain and simple, and if you enjoy eating and want to stay healthy, I believe you'll benefit from this book immensely. Bon appétit!

Kev Krueger
Cofounder, National Hepatitis C Coalition, Inc.
P.O. Box 5058
Hemet, CA 92544
National Hepline (951) 658-4414
www.nationalhepatitis-c.org

Preface

The Hepatitis C Epidemic and the Reasons for This Book

My first experience with hepatitis C was in the spring of 1998. I was twenty-seven. My fifty-one-year-old father came to visit me, and when I opened the door to receive him he fell down and passed out. I panicked, and although I only weighed 110 pounds and he weighed over 200, I somehow managed to drag him into my car and drive him to the ER. After the doctors saw him and he regained consciousness, I was told he had a severe case of hepatitis C. The doctors told me that my father was very ill and did not have long to live. That was nearly six years ago, and he is here to prove otherwise!

The intent of this book is to assist hepatitis C sufferers in living a longer and healthier life through good food management practices. Hepatitis C is not always fatal, and you can actively fight it. Similar to AIDS, this disease affects the body's immune system and pollutes the blood supply, adversely affecting the liver's functioning capacity. However, the AIDS "epidemic" is said to be smaller than what doctors expect to see from the hepatitis C virus in the future. The annual number of those infected with the hepatitis C virus is expected to exceed the number of victims claimed by the AIDS virus within the next ten years. Many people do not know they have this disease, as it can lie dormant for years and then suddenly arise. It is contracted most commonly through blood transfusions, but can also be contracted through shared needles and sexual intercourse.

If you have the virus, there are several experimental and conventional medical treatments available. However, you may not be a candidate for them, or they may not work for you, or you may just prefer a more naturalistic approach. When you are diagnosed, most doctors will give you a basic diet to follow. I will never forget the first time I heard this "basic diet" described to my very ill father and me. It was "boiled this" and "plain that." Although my father needed that type of extreme diet for the first few months after he was diagnosed, it wasn't a lifelong requirement for him. After those first few months of surviving due to extended bed rest, herbal supplements, teas, and a staunch diet, he was eager for some "real" food, instead of boiled chicken.

Eating does not have to be a miserable experience for hepatitis C sufferers. Using guidelines from the medical profession, this book will give you healthful and tasty foods to eat *and* enjoy. You can live well, even with hepatitis C. Making dietary changes can also make a significant difference in your attitude, and in the variety, severity, and frequency of your symptoms, as well as enhance the quality of your life.

• • •

We discovered that my father's blackout that day on my doorstep had probably been brought on by ingesting Tylenol (acetaminophen) for a severe headache and then drinking alcohol—the first "no-no" I learned about this disease.

I later learned that in the early '70s my father had been admitted to the hospital for "infectious hepatitis," as it was then called. Back then the medical profession did not know much about this disease, what lasting effects it would have, and how many strains would later arise. My father had been living with this disease in his body for nearly thirty years and never knew what it was doing to him! The doctors attributed the disease coming out of "remission" to an accumulation of stress from several large events that had significantly changed my father's life.

After the doctor told me that he did not expect my father to live very long and there was nothing they could do for him at that time other than suggest bed rest and a bland diet with no sugar, salt, preservatives, chemicals, or red meat, I took him home.

He was so ill that he slept for days without getting up at all. I checked on him frequently, fearing he might die. He lost his job at the family business in New York. His fiancée broke up with him because she did not want to care for an unemployed, sick husband. His future looked bleak.

I was so young—I had never thought of a parent dying, and it really upset me. I began a quest to make my father better—if he ever woke up. I studied herbs and went to organic food stores. I started a garden and grew herbs that I found were helpful to his condition, such as milk thistle, dandelion, ginger root, and green tea. When my father finally woke up, he was hungry, angry, and depressed. He did not seem to want to be alive, and although I hated to bring him bad news, I told him about his job and fiancée. He went into a deep depression, and it was a fight to get him to eat. He mostly just slept. When he did awake he would forget where he was, who he was, and that he was ill.

Over the next several months I conversed with many doctors, specialists, and other health professionals. I dragged my father to anyone I thought might be able to help him. He was only willing because he was so tired and sick. He was a different person now. He suffered from many symptoms: brain fog, muscle spasms, severe fatigue, memory loss, extreme nausea, migraine headaches, continued blackouts, paranoia, anger, confusion, jaundice, deep depression, and many others. As he regained some energy he began to talk to other hepatitis C sufferers online, and found some solace and help with Kev Krueger of the National Hepatitis C Coalition. Since he had nowhere else to go, I promised him I would be there for him until the end. He was so ill I did not think it would be a long time, and I wanted to do what I could for him.

He began seeing a therapist for his depression, and his specialist performed tests to see if he could take the experimental drugs that were available. The tests showed that he should not take the drugs. The two experimental drugs on the market at that time, Interferon and Ribovarin, had severe side effects. One of the most obvious was that some people committed suicide while on these drugs, so the medical profession began looking at their patients more carefully, screening out those they believed would have this tendency. My father fell into the projected suicide group, and his doctors believed that the risk was not worth it, besides all the other complications he had. Back to nature I went. I bought a hepa filter air cleaner for the house and ran it constantly (the humidity where I lived in the southern United States carried so many airborne allergens and germs that this was necessary), as well as a dehumidifier to prevent his weak immune system from absorbing the germs in the air. In humid climates bacteria and germs attach to the water molecules in the air, making people with weak immune systems, like those with hepatitis C, much more susceptible to illness. I made sure my father did not come into contact with people who had colds, as even the slightest interaction with someone gave him severe flu, bronchial infections, and pneumonia. I ran the air conditioner constantly during the summer, and Dad could not go outside in the yard because he was prone to heat seizures. He would be sitting in a chair and the hot humid air would get to him so quickly that he would start to convulse, his eyes rolling in his head. The first time I saw it, I found it frightening. I tried to hold him upright and keep him from falling out of his chair. He felt very hot to the touch and was sweating profusely. I ended up getting the garden hose and spraying cold water on him. He came out of the seizure fairly quickly then, and did not remember anything about it. At first I did not connect it to the heat, and neither did he or his doctors, but after this happened a few times, I made the connection. From that point on, I kept him cool, and he has not had a seizure since.

I bought only organic produce and cooked everything from scratch. It was time consuming, tiring, and frustrating. I was an unpaid nurse without a degree, on call twenty-four hours. I had no personal life. I did not receive any assistance from the government, family members, or those I thought were friends. It was a desperately dark time, but I refused to give up.

After almost a year my father was still alive and well enough to eat a greater variety of foods. I began creating recipes for him that he would enjoy and I would not have to fight to get him to eat. However, his doctors said he was still getting too many symptoms and side illnesses from so many germs, and he could not go outside or interact with people because of the danger of getting so sick that he would die of something other than the actual hepatitis C. He had also developed high levels of iron in his blood, a condition called hemochromatosis. Most people who are diagnosed with this condition have it for life. The first response is usually to stop adding iron to your diet. The second is bloodletting as a means of removing excess iron from the body. Dad did both. He went to a phlebotomist once a week for six months. I took all iron out of his diet during this time. When he went for his next blood test at the end of the six months, the hemochromatosis was gone. I added the iron slowly back into his diet in natural forms, and he has had no more problems.

My father was also so nauseous during this time that he was constantly about to vomit. He was unable to take any conventional medicines. Ginger root (a traditional antinausea remedy) no longer helped. He was not out of the woods by any means. It was suggested that I move my father to a dry environment where it might be easier for him to breathe and he would not be so susceptible to illness. The hope was that he might have a chance to function somewhat, or at least be more comfortable until the end. So we moved.

I uprooted everything in our lives and moved the two of us to the northwest, where it is dry and cool. I started all over from the ground up. I was a modern pioneer woman. I bought dry agricultural land and began building a simple cabin with the help of neighbors and new friends. I used solar for power and natural materials to build with, keeping my father's health in mind. Today we have an orchard and a vegetable garden; I also grow herbs and raise organic chicken and lamb, and we keep hens for eggs. What I cannot grow, I buy from organic food stores. I still continue to supplement my father's diet with a multivitamin, and liver-support formulas. I have changed his routine, using nature to help with time of eating and sleeping. I continue to research and learn new ways to keep him alive and getting better.

I know it's working because he is still here to prove his doctors wrong. Even after surviving that initial period, he was told he probably only had a couple of years left without a transplant. I have not been successful in getting him on the transplant list, and his doctors have advised me that a transplant would be impractical for my father (besides the prohibitive cost). Based on his overall health, the odds of him being able to accept a new organ are very low, and even if his body did accept it, at best he might have a few years before the virus takes over his body again. At his age, and with the condition of his health, they advised him to simply enjoy what time he has left. However, according to their information he should have been gone four years ago. Instead, I think his quality of life is improving every day. I know he will never be able to function like he would have if we had caught this disease before it had done so much damage to his body, but it is a testament to the healing power of the human body that he is living and enjoying life!

It is my hope that anyone who reads this book will see that following a routine of good health and a diet directed at fighting this disease can not only increase your probability of never becoming as ill as my father did but also give you the possibility of a long, fruitful life!

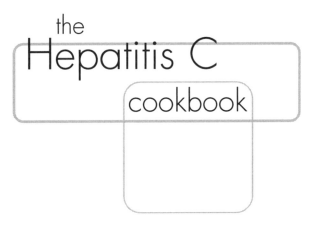

the
Hepatitis C
cookbook

Introduction

If you have hepatitis C and are either taking conventional treatments or trying natural remedies, this is the book you need by your side. We have long known the importance healthy eating plays in longevity of life and overall good health. This book helps patients follow the good eating habits that most healthcare professionals, including myself, suggest for those with this disease. Hepatitis C has long been termed the "silent epidemic" because many people who have this disease are not aware of it. It can live for years in the human body without enough symptoms to cause the patient to think about getting tested.

Hepatitis C is, however, a serious health threat. Untreated, this disease creates havoc inside your liver that can cause irreparable damage. Although there has been a rise in coverage in newspapers and new books on this subject, as well as an increased number of people getting tested, hepatitis C is still dangerous to your health if not managed. Although only about 20 percent of those who are diagnosed with hepatitis C actually proceed to cirrhosis and then death, living with this disease can be difficult, and even debilitating. This epidemic is growing faster than the expectations for a cure; in fact, the number of hepatitis C patients is expected to exceed the number of AIDS patients in just a few short years. There still is no cure for this disease and your best assault on it is to take care of your health to reduce the severity of the symptoms.

The Hepatitis C Cookbook is an excellent companion in the kitchen and on your grocery shopping trips. For long-term management of this disease, this book has you covered as well. It is written in easy-to-understand language and a simple format, so even the most basic of cooks can find recipes that they can make. The author has firsthand experience in caring for her father, who has had this disease for over thirty years, six of which have been spent completely in her care. When modern medicine could not help her father, the author used natural remedies and created recipes like the ones in this book, and by doing so she was able to bring her father back from death's door.

Eugene Somner, M.D.

1

Doctors' Guidelines for Your Diet

Although the symptoms and severity of this disease vary, there are basic guidelines most doctors give to new hepatitis C patients. And whether you opt to pursue conventional treatments or not, the dietary guidelines are important. The first rule is to cut out alcohol, period. Limit your intake of red meat, and gradually wean yourself away from it until you either don't eat it at all or eat it very infrequently. Meats are difficult to digest, taking eight to ten hours, and are usually high in fat and toxins. Avoid salt and excessive sugar. Use washed raw organic sugar or honey. Drink water, a minimum of six to eight glasses per day, to help your liver flush the toxins within it. Avoid all fast food, restaurant-prepared foods, chemicals, preservatives, and frozen prepared foods. Avoid fried foods and excessive fats. Stay away from junk food. Avoid soft drinks in general, especially those containing caffeine. Ground roasted dandelion root can substitute for and is prepared the same way as coffee. You can find organic roasted dandelion root at most natural health food stores internationally.

Use fresh and, where possible, organic fruits, vegetables, whole grains, beans, herbs, etc., even in cooking. Use distilled or spring water instead of tap water. Distilled water is recommended because all organisms are cooked out in the distillation process.

Eat frequent smaller meals five or six times in a twenty-four-hour period, rather than fewer larger meals. Take a high-quality multivitamin and ingest with food to maximize absorption. Taking a liver-support formula along with a multivitamin is a good way to help aid liver function. Most health food stores carry them. Look for formulas that contain milk thistle, dandelion root, lipioc acid, and selenium. Make sure that there are no chemicals or fillers. Everything that your liver has to process puts strain on it. If you are concerned about hemochromatosis (too much iron in the blood), then make sure you are taking a multivitamin without iron and use only low-iron packaged products. Good nutrition is very important for maintaining good health and supporting your liver's ability to help heal itself.

To increase your digestive function, chew food well and eat

under restful conditions. Do not bolt food or eat when stressed. Eating while relaxed maximizes parasympathic nervous system function and allows your body to absorb the maximum nutrient value from your food. It also helps curb digestion problems that can occur as side effects of this disease. Your largest daily meal should be eaten between noon and 2:00 p.m. This is the time when your body is at its optimum, and thus the most opportune period to digest a large meal. Following this schedule will make digesting a full meal easier on your body and liver functions.

Bitter foods can assist in alleviating nausea, as well as catnip, ginger root, and licorice root teas. Eat cool foods such as fresh salads and sandwiches, and eat small amounts. Drinking ginger ale can also help.

If you experience diarrhea, eat raw, peeled apples, which contain pectin.

Following your doctor's dietary guidelines and the hints in this book will reduce or eliminate gastric reflux. However, if you experience gastric symptoms even when you avoid highly spiced foods and caffeinated drinks, stay upright for thirty minutes after eating.

Should you become constipated, remember to drink plenty of water and eat prunes or drink prune juice. Try to keep yourself from developing constipation because it is very hard on your body and liver to have the poisons and toxins inside. The longer they remain in your body, the more they will negatively impact how you feel.

Eliminating toxins and toxin buildup is important for everyone. However, for those with hepatitis C, this can be critical to how you feel from day to day. As your body builds up toxins, your liver and other organs become sluggish and your symptoms can increase in both severity and longevity. This has been a vital part of my father's survival. In order to keep toxins from building up, he must continually eliminate them. Keeping your bowel movements regular and easy is an important factor and can be facilitated by remembering to drink plenty of distilled water throughout the day. By following the tips in this book and changing your diet, you will also make sure that fewer toxins enter your body, thus ensuring that your body will not be forced to work as hard to get rid of them. Remember that your liver is your body's filter and that like the filter on your air conditioner, it gets dirty. The more you run your air conditioner, the more dirt its filter collects. If you do not clean or replace the filter, side effects begin to occur: the machinery becomes less efficient and works harder to perform, your electric bill increases, fewer germs and allergens will be removed, and your air will remain contaminated. It is the same for your liver. If you keep your liver's environment clean, it will be able to function better. You can actually help your liver to heal itself by caring for it. The disease will still progress, but you can slow it, and keep your liver regenerating itself.

2

Buying the Right Foods

Besides just eating well, choosing the best foods can also make a difference in how you feel. I experimented with my father considerably, researching labels, brands, prices, and his reactions to what he ate. Typically the highest quality items will be more expensive, but consider what you are getting and what you can afford. You can use canned, frozen, dry, or fresh products in all the recipes in this book, but I strongly recommend using fresh products whenever possible. In fact, I have had the most success with using organic products. However, it's a good idea to read the labels, because even they can have additives.

Produce is best bought fresh, used fresh, and purchased at organic stores, farmers markets, or roadside stands. If you make it a habit to use what's in season, some supermarkets will carry locally grown produce too. When in doubt, ask. Wherever possible use fresh fruits and vegetables versus canned or frozen items. At the back of this book you will find an appendix listing some great resources for natural or organic products.

Get in the habit of reading all labels. Many products vary in amounts of sodium and preservatives. You can find products with low amounts, and these will do when you just don't have the time to cook full meals from scratch. I do suggest, however, taking the extra time out of your day to create good meals like those outlined in this book.

Another option is to grow some produce yourself, such as vegetables and herbs. I have found gardening to be quite therapeutic, and it gives you the best possible freshness and taste, not to mention the obvious cost benefits. When it comes to taking care of yourself, it is well worth the effort.

Many vegetables and herbs can be grown in pots outdoors, even in small spaces, or indoors in some cases. Tomatoes can be grown well in pots, and can be brought inside and grown in a warm sunny location during winter months. Tomatoes are also often disappointing in grocery stores and very pricey in organic food markets. The reason is that the tomatoes are not typically vine ripened; in order to transport them across the country, they are picked green and put into dark rooms where they are exposed to ethylene gas. This forces the tomatoes to turn red, but they are not ripe, so the taste is lacking. Many times I've bought a beautiful healthy-looking tomato, only to go home and slice it for a cold antipasto dish or salad and find that it was not tasty at all. Additionally many people make the mistake of storing tomatoes in the refrigerator. Tomatoes should never be stored under 50°F, and should be used off the vine right away. Growing your own gives you everything you could ask for in a tomato. Try it!

Other vegetables that can easily be grown in small spaces or pots are lettuces, bush type cucumbers, eggplant, peppers, and bush type beans. These grow well on decks, patios, and in small yards.

Herbs are a large category with much to offer. My first experimenting with herbs was for my father and included calendula, catnip, dandelion, milk thistle, and valerian. As I began to change his diet I realized the value of seasoning with other herbs for flavor and texture. Any of the herbs used in the recipes in this book can be easily grown in beds, in a small yard, or in pots. Some herbs, such as chives, parsley, oregano, rosemary, and basil, can be grown in small pots indoors year-round in a sunny window. I grow a great variety of culinary and medicinal herbs during the summer. In their growing season I use them fresh, and then I dry the rest of the harvest for use during the winter months. I wash the plants in place, allow to air dry, and then trim off what I want and lay flat on trays. I store them in a cool, dark place until they are dried, then crumble and store in labeled jars. I store them out of direct light and their flavor lasts all winter, until my plants come up again in the spring.

Remember to eat something every three to four hours during the day, and to eat your main meal between noon and 2:00 p.m. whenever possible for optimal digestion.

Another important dietary guideline involves combining different types of food. Don't eat meat and dairy products at the same meal. Chicken alfredo may be tasty, but it is very hard for the body to digest and process both dairy and meat at the same time. You can use dairy products for flavoring, but avoid cream and cheese sauces on meats.

If you have any concerns about elevated iron, do not use any cast-iron cookware. Food cooked in cast-iron pans always absorbs some iron.

Vegetables like broccoli, Brussels sprouts, cabbage, and cauliflower are especially good for you and contain sulfur, which is important for the production of proteins in the liver. When cooking fresh produce, never boil it or overcook (soft or mushy). Use a small amount of water in the bottom of your pan and steam the vegetables. You want to preserve all the nutrients you can.

When using dairy products choose those with low or reduced fat. If dairy aggravates your system, try goat's milk or soy milk.

Do not use artificial sweeteners unless your doctor instructs otherwise. Use washed raw organic sugar or honey and use even these sparingly. Both of these items can be found in most grocery stores, as well as health food markets. When picking honey, look for raw, organic honey, not honey that has been "cut" with Karo syrup. Organic honey is safe because even if bees feed on plants that have been fertilized or sprayed the toxins are eliminated in the process of producing their honey. It's one of nature's marvels. If your natural honey crystallizes, don't fret, just place the jar in hot (not boiling) water it until the honey "melts," then use. Cooking honey destroys the many nutrients in it and affects its taste as well.

When using a fat, use olive oil, unsalted butter, or ghee. They are natural and have the best value. Again, buy the best quality you can. Do not try new fat substitutes like olestra, because they can cause or aggravate gastrointestinal problems, including cramping and diarrhea.

Now you are ready to begin making yourself feel better. Let's get cooking!

3

Breakfast

You have no doubt heard that breakfast is the most important meal of the day. However, for sufferers of hepatitis C, mornings can come with considerable nausea. Do not give up on breakfast, but try eating after you have had a glass of water and freshly squeezed orange juice, have eliminated toxins, and are fully awake. You should take your vitamins and medication with breakfast as well. I have marked recipes in this chapter that have been particularly helpful in easing my father's nausea.

Quarter-Slice Melon

This recipe is good for those who wake up very nauseous.

1   whole ripe organic sweet honeydew melon

Organic ginger root, grated or powdered

Slice the melon in half, then in half again so that you have four quarters. Using a sharp knife cut the melon under the flesh close to the rind from one end to the other. Then cut the melon flesh lengthwise. Cut the melon down to the rind crosswise, leaving the chunks in place on the rind. Sprinkle the ginger root on the melon. Let sit in the refrigerator for 1 hour. Serve cold or heat in the microwave for 30 seconds and serve.

Serves 4

Atole (Cornmeal Porridge)

This breakfast dates back to pre-Hispanic times and is considered a comfort food—often given to the elderly, sick, and new mothers because of its ease on the body's digestive system. It can also be served as a drink by adding more milk.

¾　cup blue cornmeal

½　cup plus 2 tablespoons cold
　　distilled water

1　cup 2 percent milk

4　pats unsalted butter

　　Raw organic sugar

In a large saucepan bring 2 cups of water to a boil. In a medium bowl mix the cornmeal with the cold distilled water to form a soft paste. Whisking constantly, pour the cornmeal into the boiling water. It may spit as you stir, so be cautious. Reduce the heat to low and cook for 8 to 10 minutes, until thick. In a small saucepan heat the milk until bubbles form around the inside edge. Pour the atole into 4 bowls. Place 1 pat of butter on top of the atole and sprinkle with sugar. Pour milk over each portion and serve warm.

Serves 4

Italian Two-Egg Omelet

1	tablespoon organic unsalted butter
2	farm fresh eggs
2	tablespoons low fat milk
2	tablespoons leftover homemade tomato sauce
1	organic melrose or ¼ green bell pepper, chopped
1	teaspoon dried organic oregano or ½ teaspoon fresh
1	teaspoon dried tarragon or ½ teaspoon fresh
1	pinch white pepper
1½	teaspoons freeze-dried chives or 1 teaspoon fresh
1	large or two small slices Swiss cheese
	Sprinkle of Parmesan cheese

In a skillet melt the butter on medium heat. In a medium bowl mix the eggs, milk, tomato sauce, melrose or bell pepper, oregano, tarragon, white pepper, and chives. Beat well, and pour into the skillet. Reduce the heat, and with a nonstick spatula keep the edges from sticking to the pan. Lay the slice(s) of Swiss cheese across the middle. When the cheese is melted, the omelet is ready. Slide and fold onto a plate. Sprinkle with Parmesan cheese and serve warm.

Serves 1 to 2

Honey French Toast

Can help relieve nausea.

½ cup raw organic honey, plus more
    for drizzling
1 cup 2 percent milk
6 farm fresh eggs
1½ teaspoons cinnamon
1 teaspoon ginger
12 thick slices French bread
    Organic unsalted butter
    Toasted pecan pieces

In a large bowl beat together the honey, milk, eggs, cinnamon, and ginger. Dip the bread slices in the egg mixture, turning to coat. In a skillet melt the butter and brown the soaked bread slices over medium heat, turning once. Drizzle honey over the toast and sprinkle with pecans.

Serves 6

Herbed Scrambled Eggs

4	farm fresh eggs
1	tablespoon 2 percent milk
1	tablespoon chopped fresh parsley
1	tablespoon chopped fresh chives
1	tablespoon chopped fresh tarragon
½	medium onion, finely chopped
1	to 2 tablespoons unsalted butter

In a small bowl mix the eggs, milk, parsley, chives, tarragon, and onion. In a skillet melt the butter, then pour in the egg mixture. Turn the eggs occasionally with a spatula until cooked. Serve immediately.

Serves 2

Egg Tortilla

Pico de Gallo sauce:

1   large tomato, chopped
½   medium onion, chopped
1   teaspoon cilantro, chopped

1   to 2 tablespoons unsalted butter
4   farm fresh eggs
2   flour tortillas
    Shredded Cheddar cheese
    Low-sodium sour cream (optional)
    Fresh chopped parsley or cilantro
    for garnish

To make the Pico de Gallo sauce, in a medium bowl mix the tomato, onion, and cilantro. Set aside.

In a medium skillet heat the butter. Prepare the eggs sunny side up. Heat the tortillas, if desired, in the oven until warm, or use at room temperature. Place two eggs on each tortilla. Top with Pico de Gallo sauce, shredded Cheddar cheese, sour cream (if desired), and parsley or cilantro. Serve immediately.

Serves 2

Strawberry Crêpes with Honey Sauce

Honey Sauce:

½ cup raw organic honey

⅓ cup fresh-squeezed orange juice

1 tablespoon fresh-squeezed lemon juice

2 teaspoons grated orange peel

1 teaspoon grated lemon peel

1½ teaspoons cornstarch

1 tablespoon unsalted butter

Crêpes:

2 cups 2 percent milk

1 cup organic unbleached flour

2 egg yolks

1 whole egg

1 tablespoon raw organic honey

1 tablespoon olive oil

2 cups sliced fresh ripe strawberries

First, make the sauce. In a small saucepan whisk the honey, juices, peels, and cornstarch until well blended and the cornstarch is dissolved. Bring the mixture to a boil over medium-high heat. Whisking frequently, cook until the mixture thickens. Remove. Whisk in the butter. Set aside and let cool to room temperature.

To make the crêpes, combine the milk, flour, egg yolks, egg, 1 tablespoon honey, and olive oil in a blender or food processor. Process until smooth. Rub an 8-inch skillet with a paper towel dipped in olive oil. Heat over medium-high heat. Spoon 3 to 4 tablespoons batter into the skillet, rotating until the skillet is covered evenly with batter. Cook until the edges start to brown. Turn the crêpe over and cook until lightly browned. Remove to a plate and cool. Cook the remaining crêpes. (Can be refrigerated for three days or frozen for up to 1 month.)

To assemble, put sliced strawberries on one half of each crêpe, fold over, and top with sauce. Serve immediately.

Serves 6

Ginger Muffins

Can help nausea.

1	1- to 2-ounce piece unpeeled organic ginger root
¾	cup plus 3 tablespoons raw organic sugar
2	tablespoons fresh lemon zest, with some pith attached
1	stick or ½ cup unsalted butter at room temperature
2	farm fresh eggs
1	cup 2 percent milk
2	cups organic unbleached flour
¾	teaspoon baking soda

Preheat the oven to 375°F. Grease the tins of a muffin pan. In a food processor grate the ginger into tiny pieces. In a small skillet cook the ginger and ¼ cup sugar over medium heat. Do not leave unattended, as sugar melts quickly. When the sugar is completely melted and is hot, remove from the heat and cool.

In the food processor combine the lemon zest and 3 tablespoons sugar, grating into tiny bits. Add to the ginger mixture, mix thoroughly, and set aside.

In a large mixing bowl beat the butter. Add ½ cup sugar, and beat until smooth. Add the eggs, and beat well. Add the milk, and blend. Add the flour and baking soda next, beating until the mixture is smooth. Finally, add the lemon-ginger mixture and blend thoroughly.

Spoon the batter into the muffin tins so that each section is three-fourths full. Bake for 15 to 20 minutes. Remove from the pan to a wire rack and serve warm.

Makes 16 muffins

Potatoes & Eggs

2   to 3 tablespoons unsalted butter
    or ghee
1   pound red potatoes, diced into
    ¾-inch pieces
1   large onion, chopped
8   farm fresh eggs
    Fresh ground pepper to taste

In a large skillet melt the butter over medium heat. Add the potatoes, stirring occasionally, and cook for about 8 minutes, until half cooked. Add the onion and cook for another 8 minutes, until the potatoes and onions are soft. Beat the eggs and pour into the potato mixture. Heat, stirring constantly, for about 5 minutes, until the eggs are set. Sprinkle with pepper and serve.

Serves 4

Organic Granola Cereal

Organic granola
2 percent milk (optional)
Fruit (optional)

In a single-serving bowl add milk and/or fruit to organic granola. Blend well and serve.

Serves 1

Semolina Cereal

¼   cup semolina
1   cup water
1   tablespoon unsalted butter
¼   teaspoon ground cinnamon
3   tablespoons raw organic sugar
1   cup 2 percent milk

In a saucepan cook the semolina in the water until fully combined. Add the butter, cinnamon, sugar, and milk, and stir to blend. Cook on medium heat for approximately 20 minutes, until the mixture has the consistency of pudding. Add more milk if you desire a smoother consistency. For thicker cereal, add more semolina. Serve.

Serves 1

4

The Main Meal: Dinner

In many cultures eating the main meal in the middle of the day is still practiced. In the United States, because of our hectic work schedules, lunch has become a smaller meal, often eaten hastily, and we reserve our main meal for when we get home, usually not until 6:00 p.m. or later. Scientifically, it is known that our bodies are best able to digest a large meal during midday, usually between the hours of noon and 2:00 p.m. I tried this with my father and definitely noticed less nausea and other digestive problems when he followed this regimen.

Turkey Burgers

1 ½ pounds organic ground turkey
1 tablespoon organic garlic powder
1 tablespoon onion powder
1 tablespoon dried parsley
White pepper to taste
2 slices organic/homemade whole grain bread
1 fresh pineapple

In a large bowl combine the ground turkey, garlic powder, onion powder, parsley, and white pepper. Divide and form into 4 patties, and cook on a hot griddle or grill using no additional fat. Cook thoroughly. Remove from the heat. Place each patty on a bread slice. Remove the outer skin of the pineapple, core, and make thick slices. Place a slice of pineapple on top of each turkey burger. Serve.

Serves 4

Shredded Potatoes

4   medium to large organic baking
    potatoes
1   pint light cream
    White pepper
8   ounces sharp Cheddar cheese,
    grated

Preheat the oven to 300°F. Wash and shred the potatoes using a grater. Place the grated potatoes in a large microwave-safe bowl of cold water. Microwave on high for 10 minutes, checking at 8 minutes. Strain and rinse. Put the potatoes back in the bowl. Add the cream and pepper, and mix thoroughly. Pour into an 8 x 8-inch baking dish. Sprinkle the grated Cheddar cheese on top of the potatoes. Bake until the cheese is fully melted and the edges are crisp, approximately 20 minutes. Remove from the oven and cool slightly before serving.

Serves 4

Italiano Pie

Crust:

2¼ cups organic flour, plus extra for rolling

¾ cup extra-virgin olive oil from Italy

⅓ cup distilled water

1 farm fresh egg

Filling:

3 tablespoons extra-virgin olive oil

2 cloves organic garlic, minced

2 onions, thinly sliced

3 small organic or farm-raised eggplant

White pepper to taste

1 teaspoon chopped fresh thyme

6 ripe, fresh, organic or homegrown tomatoes, thinly sliced

Preheat the oven to 425°F. In a large bowl or a food processor combine the flour, ¾ cup olive oil, water, and egg. When the dough forms a ball, wrap it in plastic and refrigerate for 1 hour.

In a large skillet heat 3 tablespoons olive oil over medium heat, then sauté the garlic and onions until soft and fragrant.

Add the eggplant. Cook until it softens, approximately 8 minutes. Add the pepper and thyme, and set aside to cool.

Roll the dough out on a floured surface to about ¼-inch thickness. Line a 9-inch springform or quiche pan with the dough. Cover the dough with parchment paper and use pastry weights to hold down. Bake for 10 minutes and then remove the paper and weights. Fill the crust with the eggplant mixture, alternating with the sliced tomatoes in a circular fashion. Bake for 18 minutes. Serve warm.

Serves 6

Amish Herb Noodles

Noodles:

3   farm fresh eggs

2   cups flour

2   to 3 tablespoons fresh chopped chives

1   to 2 tablespoons fresh chopped parsley

Fresh ground pepper to taste

In a large bowl beat the eggs until they froth. Add the flour slowly until a dough is created. Knead the dough smooth. Turn the dough out onto a floured surface and roll out, turning often, to ⅛-inch thickness. Allow to dry for 45 minutes, turn, and dry for another 30 minutes. Using a pizza cutter or a sharp knife, cut the dough into noodle strips.

In a large saucepan boil water over high heat. Add the noodles and stir. Cook for about 10 minutes, stirring often, until the noodles are tender but still firm. Drain the noodles and set aside ½ cup of the cooking water. Return the noodles to the pan. Add the chives, parsley, and the reserved water. Over high heat toss the noodles until all of the liquid is absorbed. Season with fresh pepper and serve warm.

Serves 4

Asparagus Penne

1	pound penne pasta
1	to 2 pounds homegrown or organic asparagus
¼	cup extra-virgin olive oil
4	scallions, chopped
1	tablespoon unsalted butter
3	cloves garlic, thinly sliced

Bring a large pot of water to a boil, then add the pasta and cook until almost al dente (firm, but not hard). Drain, reserving ½ cup of the cooking water. Wash and cut on an angle the best of each asparagus spear. In a large skillet heat the olive oil and add the scallions. Sauté until soft, about 3 minutes. Add the asparagus and butter, and cook for 8 minutes, until fork-tender. Add the garlic and cook until it wilts and the aroma escapes. Add the pasta and the reserved cooking water to the skillet. Cook for 1 minute, toss, and serve.

Serves 4

Paella

4	boneless, skinless organic chicken breasts, fat trimmed
1	tablespoon onion powder
1	tablespoon cumin
1	tablespoon garlic powder
1	tablespoon dried oregano
2	to 3 tablespoons olive oil
2	medium onions, coarsely chopped
½	each green, yellow, and red bell pepper, chopped
4	cloves garlic, sliced
2	tablespoons chopped fresh parsley
1	14.5-ounce can low-salt diced tomatoes
3	cups Lundberg organic sweet rice or other fat rice
3	cups distilled water
2	teaspoons paprika
1	teaspoon saffron, preferably stamens, but powder will work
	Fresh or steamed peas for top

Wash, trim, and cut the chicken into large chunks. In a small bowl blend the onion powder, cumin, garlic powder, and oregano. Coat the chicken with the mixture. Set aside.

In a flat-bottomed pan or large skillet heat the olive oil and cook the onions, bell pepper, garlic, and parsley on medium-high heat until wilted, about 10 minutes. Push the vegetables to the sides of the pan and add the chicken to the center. Cook, but not fully. Remove the chicken (if using a pot, remove the vegetables to cook the chicken, then remove the chicken and re-add the vegetables). Add the tomatoes. Blend and warm. Add the rice and stir, mixing well. Add the distilled water and stir. Add the paprika and saffron, and simmer, covered, for a few minutes, until the water thickens. Add the chicken, blending, and let the mixture cook until slow bubbles form. To get the traditional Paella crunch, let the mixture cook for an extra 40 seconds. Paella rice should be al dente (firm, but not hard). Top with fresh or steamed peas, and let stand for 10 minutes before serving.

Serves 4

Stuffed Tomatoes

6   large ripe organic tomatoes, tops
    cut and seeded

3   cups dried mushrooms (morels,
    shitake, oyster, button)

2   cups stock (vegetable, chicken,
    turkey)

1   cup hot water

1   tablespoon extra-virgin organic
    olive oil

1   medium sweet organic onion,
    chopped

1   cup homemade breadcrumbs from
    a stale bread

1   bay leaf, rough crushed

On a paper towel turn the cut and seeded tomatoes upside down to drain some juice off. In a bowl combine the 3 cups of dried mushrooms with the stock and hot water. Let sit until the mushrooms are reconstituted. In a saucepan heat the olive oil and sauté the onion until wilted and translucent. Add the bread-crumbs and bay leaf. Heat through. Squeeze the excess liquid from the mushrooms and chop. Add to the saucepan. Mix well and heat thoroughly. Place a Silpat mat on a baking sheet or lightly coat with olive oil. Turn on the broiler. Place the tomatoes on the prepared baking sheet and stuff with the mushroom mixture. Broil for about 5 minutes. Cool slightly and serve.

Serves 6

Spinach-Stuffed Chicken Breast

2 bunches fresh spinach
2 tablespoons olive oil
4 cloves garlic, crushed
¼ cup pine nuts (pignoli)
¼ cup raisins
4 large chicken breasts
2 tablespoons butter, softened
¼ cup mixture of chopped fresh parsley, oregano, and thyme

Preheat the oven to 350°F. Clean and cut the spinach. In a skillet heat the olive oil and cook the spinach. As it wilts, add the garlic. Cook through. Set aside to cool. Add the pine nuts and raisins, and blend. Stuff the chicken breasts with the spinach mixture, fold, and use toothpicks to secure. In a bowl combine the softened butter and fresh herbs; mix. Coat the chicken breasts with the herb mixture and put in a glass baking dish. Bake for at least 30 minutes, depending on the size of the breasts. To check for doneness, make a slice in the thickest part of the breast, and if the inside is still pink, cook longer.

Tip: Always allow meat to sit for 15 to 20 minutes once it's out of the oven. The meat will continue to cook as it begins cooling and the flavor and ease of cutting will be heightened as well.

Serves 4

Pasta Fungii

2   to 4 tablespoons unsalted butter

4   cloves garlic, sliced

1   small package button mushrooms, sliced

1   small package portabella mushrooms, sliced

1   pound farfalle (bow tie) low-sodium organic pasta

2   to 4 tablespoons extra-virgin olive oil

Parmesan cheese (optional)

Fresh ground pepper (optional)

In a large skillet over medium heat melt the butter and sauté the garlic until the aroma escapes, then add the sliced mushrooms. Cover and cook out the water. Then uncover and sauté the mushrooms. In a large saucepan cook the farfalle according to package directions until al dente (firm, but not hard). Drain—do not rinse—and place in a large bowl. Add the sautéed mushroom mixture. Add Parmesan cheese and/or fresh ground pepper, if desired, and toss. Serve.

Tip: The more gently you handle garlic the sweeter the flavor; the rougher you are with it the hotter it gets.

Serves 4

Turkey Chili

2	tablespoons olive oil
2	pounds organic ground turkey
1	large onion, chopped
2	teaspoons paprika
1	teaspoon cayenne pepper
4	cloves garlic, chopped
1	teaspoon chili powder
4	cups turkey stock
1	cup distilled water
1	24-ounce large can tomatoes
2	15-ounce cans organic red kidney beans, drained of liquid

In a large stockpot heat the olive oil. Add the ground turkey and cook over medium heat, breaking up clumps gently so the meat does not become tough. Add the chopped onion and cook until the meat is browned and the onions are clear and glossy. Drain off the excess fat. Add the paprika, cayenne pepper, garlic, and chili powder. Blend. Add the stock, water, and tomatoes. Cover and simmer gently for about 1 hour. Taste. Add additional spices to taste, if desired, and then add the beans. Heat through and serve.

Serves 4

No-Fry Oven Chicken

½ teaspoon cayenne pepper

1 teaspoon oregano

Fresh ground pepper to taste

1 teaspoon garlic powder

1 teaspoon onion powder

½ teaspoon marjoram

Low-sodium crackers, blended in food processor to crumbs

1 farm fresh egg plus 1 egg white

4 medium chicken breasts, deboned and skinned

Preheat the oven to 400°F. Line a baking sheet with a Silpat mat or lightly coat with butter. In a shallow dish blend the cayenne pepper, oregano, pepper, garlic powder, onion powder, marjoram, and crackers. In a small bowl beat the egg and egg white. Dredge the chicken in the spice mixture and coat well. Dip the chicken in the egg to coat, and then dredge in the spice mixture again. Place the chicken on the prepared baking sheet and bake for approximately 15 minutes, until the centers are cooked but still moist. Remove from the oven and let sit for 10 minutes before serving.

Serves 4

Cauliflower

1   large head cauliflower
4   tablespoons unsalted butter
½   cup breadcrumbs made from stale
    bread
    Fresh ground pepper to taste

Cut up the cauliflower into bite-sized florets. In a stockpot heat some distilled water and steam the cauliflower until fork-tender. Set aside. In a skillet melt the butter and add the breadcrumbs. Heat through. Pour the cauliflower into a serving bowl and pour the breadcrumbs on top. Season with ground pepper. Serve warm.

Serves 4

Turkey Meatloaf

1	pound 6 ounces lean organic ground turkey
1	tablespoon minced garlic
1	tablespoon onion flakes
2	teaspoons oregano
1	teaspoon hot (or regular) paprika
1	tablespoon lemon juice
¼	cup raw organic honey
2	tablespoons raw organic sugar
¼	cup fine plain breadcrumbs
⅛	cup pine nuts (pignoli)
2	eggs
¼	cup raisins
½	cup oats

Preheat the oven to 350°F. In a large bowl combine all of the ingredients. Mix until well blended. Transfer the mixture into mini loaf tins or muffin tins, or one large meatloaf tin. Cook. The small tins will cook in approximately 30 minutes; the large tin will take 1 hour. Remove from the oven and allow to rest before serving.

Serves 4

Dutch Casserole

10	medium baking potatoes
	Milk
4	tablespoons unsalted butter
1	medium onion, chopped
½	cup diced celery
2	cups stale bread, chopped
2	eggs, beaten
2	tablespoons chopped fresh parsley
	Fresh ground pepper to taste

Peel the potatoes. In a large stockpot place the potatoes and enough water to cover. Boil until tender.

Preheat the oven to 350°F. Drain and mash the potatoes, adding milk until the mixture is the desired consistency. Set aside. In a medium skillet over medium heat melt the butter and sauté the onion and celery. In a large bowl combine the bread, eggs, parsley, and some milk. Toss, then add the vegetable sauté and blend well. Add this mixture to the potatoes and blend. Add milk if needed to keep moist, then add the pepper. Pour into a glass baking dish and bake until golden.

Serves 4

Dutch-Style Braised Leeks

2 pounds leeks
2½ tablespoons unsalted butter
2 tablespoons unbleached flour
1 cup 2 percent milk
1 tablespoon white vinegar
Fresh ground pepper to taste

Clean the leeks and remove the ends and outer leaves. Cut into 2-inch lengths. In a large saucepan cook the leeks in water until tender, but not mushy, about 20 minutes. Drain. In a small saucepan melt the butter. Add the flour and stir until blended, then make a sauce by adding the milk and blending well. Add the vinegar and pepper. Add the leeks and cook for 10 minutes, then serve.

Serves 4

Shepherd's Pie

1	quart vegetable or chicken stock
¼	cup unbleached flour
½	cup distilled water
10	ounces pearl onions, peeled
1½	pounds potatoes, peeled and chopped
½	ounce button mushrooms, sliced
1	to 1½ pounds chicken or turkey, chopped or shredded
1½	cups sweet baby peas
2	large carrots, chopped
1	stalk celery, chopped
¾	cup 2 percent milk, heated
4	tablespoons unsalted butter
1	large egg yolk
1	teaspoon chopped fresh or dried parsley
	Fresh ground pepper to taste

Preheat the oven to 350°F. In a large stockpot bring the stock to a boil. In a small bowl combine the flour with the distilled water to make a slurry, then add to the stock and blend. Whisk to keep smooth. Add the onions, bring to a simmer, and cook for 30 minutes. In a separate pot boil the potatoes until tender.

Add the mushrooms to the sauce, then add the meat, peas, carrots, and celery. Simmer, then pour into a glass dish. Mash the potatoes and add the milk, butter, egg yolk, and parsley. Add pepper, then spread the potatoes over the stew in the dish, making a smooth surface. Bake for 20 to 25 minutes. Allow to cool slightly before serving.

Serves 4

5

Supper

Now that you have rearranged your eating schedule so that your heavier meals are earlier in the day, your evening meal will need to be made up of lighter fare so that your body can digest the food easily before you go to bed. It is not a good idea to go to bed on a full stomach because this is hard on your system. Eating lighter, smaller meals later in the day will help you sleep better and will reduce your nausea in the morning when you awake. The best time for supper is about five hours before bedtime. You can still have a small snack before retiring, like some fruit, to maintain the every-three-to-four-hour eating schedule previously discussed. The best choices for the evening meal include sandwiches, wraps, light salads, and bowls of lighter soups. Do not choose a dairy-based soup for this meal—dairy products put a strain on your system and take a long time to digest. Instead, stick with light broths and vegetable blends.

Fish Sandwich

4 pieces halibut (catfish works well also)
  Olive oil
  Paprika
  Fresh ground pepper
  Lemon
4 sandwich rolls

Preheat your outdoor or indoor grill. Drizzle one side of the fish with olive oil and season with paprika and fresh ground pepper. Place the fish on the grill surface, seasoned side down. Drizzle oil over the fish and season the second side. Flip and grill the second side. Remove from the grill and place on rolls. Squeeze fresh lemon juice over the fish. Serve as is, or add a dollop of homemade Tartar Sauce (see recipe on the next page).

Serves 4

Tartar Sauce

1 teaspoon chopped fresh chives
1 teaspoon chopped fresh dill weed
2 tablespoons finely chopped onion
1 teaspoon lemon juice
1 cup mayonnaise
2 tablespoons pickle relish

In a small bowl combine all of the ingredients. Serve with fish.

Makes enough for 4 sandwiches

Roasted Pepper Sandwich

There are many ways to roast peppers. This recipe is from my Italian-American grandmother, who learned from her immigrant mother, who adapted the recipe from her mother, who learned to cook in the homeland of Northern Italy. These can be made ahead, and in fact taste best if prepared this way.

6	large red sweet peppers
1	teaspoon dried basil
1	teaspoon dried oregano (Italian)
4	cloves garlic, sliced
¼	cup extra-virgin olive oil
	Fresh ground pepper to taste

Preheat the oven to 350°F. Rinse the peppers. Place in a large roasting pan. Put in the oven and watch carefully. When the bottom side shows partially black, turn. Repeat until all sides have been scorched and the skin is loose, approximately 45 minutes. Remove the peppers and cover with a damp cloth, allowing them to cool enough to handle and make the skins easier to take off. Take the stems and cores out by hand. Gently pour the inside juices (don't worry if some seeds get in) into a large bowl. Peel the peppers and then rip them into thin slices. When all of the peppers are done and in the bowl, add the basil, oregano, garlic, olive oil, and fresh ground pepper, and blend. Allow to stand for 30 minutes, then refrigerate for at least 1 hour. If serving the next day, take out of the refrigerator about 30 minutes before serving. Serve on Italian bread.

Serves 4

Egg Salad Sandwich

6 organic farm fresh eggs

½ onion, finely chopped

1 stalk celery, finely chopped (optional)

½ teaspoon paprika

Fresh ground pepper to taste

¼ cup (or less if desired) mayonnaise

In a saucepan boil the eggs for 4 minutes. Cool and peel. The eggs should not have a fully hard center. Chop finely and place in a bowl. Add the onion, celery (if desired), paprika, pepper, and mayonnaise, and blend to the desired consistency. Spread on any type of bread and serve.

Serves 2

Lemongrass, Spinach, and Mushroom Soup

5	cups distilled water
4	ounces rice sticks
1	cup vegetable stock
4	scallions (green onions), thinly chopped
¼	cup finely chopped fresh lemongrass
1	package button mushrooms, sliced
2	tablespoons grated fresh ginger
3	cups cut up fresh spinach, stems removed
	Fresh ground pepper to taste

Heat the distilled water. In a large bowl soak the rice sticks in the hot distilled water until soft. Drain and set aside. In a large pot combine the stock, scallions, lemongrass, mushrooms, ginger, and drained rice sticks. Simmer for about 3 minutes. Remove from the heat and add the spinach. Stir well. Let sit a few minutes before serving. Add fresh ground pepper.

Serves 4

Stuffed Peppers

½ cup distilled water
¾ cup vegetable stock
½ cup quick-cook barley
1 tablespoon olive oil
1 cup sliced button mushrooms
½ medium onion, finely chopped
2 large sweet bell peppers of any
   color
1 egg
1 large ripe tomato, cut into small
   chunks
½ teaspoon dried rosemary
½ teaspoon dried basil
½ teaspoon dried oregano
3 tablespoons breadcrumbs
   Fresh ground pepper to taste

Preheat the oven to 350°F. In a large saucepan combine the water, stock, and barley, and bring to a boil over medium heat. Simmer, covered, for 10 minutes or until the barley is tender. Drain any excess liquid and set aside. In a saucepan heat the olive oil and sauté the mushrooms and onion. Set aside when the liquid from the mushrooms is gone and the onions are clear and soft. Cut the tops off the peppers, core, and remove the seeds.

In a saucepan cook the peppers in boiling water for 2 minutes. Drain and set aside. In a bowl stir together the egg, tomato, herbs, breadcrumbs, and the mushroom and onion mixture, and blend. Add the barley and scoop into the peppers. Sprinkle fresh pepper on top. Set the peppers in a roasting pan and bake, covered with aluminum foil, for approximately 30 minutes, until the filling is fully heated. Let cool slightly before serving.

Serves 2

Ranchera Soup

3 quarts chicken stock

2 large garlic cloves, peeled and sliced in half lengthwise

1 medium onion, diced

2 large ripe tomatoes, diced

½ cup coursely chopped cilantro (fresh only)

1 cup shredded cooked chicken

2 ripe avocados, diced

Fresh ground pepper to taste

1 lime, cut into wedges (optional)

In a large pot combine the chicken stock and garlic cloves. On high heat, bring to a boil for 1 minute, then simmer, partially covered, for 1 hour. Remove the garlic. While keeping the soup simmering, add the onion and cook for 5 to 6 minutes. Add the tomatoes, cilantro, and chicken. Simmer a few more minutes. Let the soup rest for a few minutes. Top each bowl with diced avocado and ground pepper. Squirt lime juice on top, if desired.

Serves 6

Linguine Soup

2 quarts chicken stock

10 ounces dried linguine (break into smaller pieces if desired)

6 sprigs fresh marjoram, chopped

3 farm fresh eggs

Fresh ground pepper to taste

Parmesan cheese to taste

In a large pot bring the stock to a boil. Add the linguine and marjoram. Return to a boil. Cook until the pasta is al dente (firm, but not hard). Meanwhile, in a medium bowl beat the eggs well and add 2 tablespoons of broth from the soup. Mix well. When the pasta is cooked stir in the egg mixture. Ladle into bowls and top the soup with ground pepper and Parmesan cheese.

Serves 4

Sweet Indian Rice

This is wonderful aromatic rice dish that goes well with all kinds of cuisine, or as here, is just a nice light meal in itself. Some tips when making this rice are:

1. *Always rinse the rice 6 times.*
2. *Soak the rice for 30 minutes.*
3. *Fully drain the rice for 20 minutes before cooking.*
4. *Use very low heat to cook the rice.*
5. *Use aluminum foil to completely seal the pot while the rice is cooking.*
6. *Never open the lid when the rice is cooking to check it.*
7. *Always use a slotted spoon to gently dish out the rice so that the grains do not break.*

½	teaspoon saffron threads
2	tablespoons warm 2 percent milk
1	cup Basmati rice
4	tablespoons unsalted butter or ghee
4	whole cardamom pods
1	stick cinnamon
1⅓	cups distilled water
¾	teaspoon turmeric
5	whole cloves
3	bay leaves
2	tablespoons raisins

In a small skillet heat the saffron over medium heat. Stir until the saffron is a few shades darker, then remove from the heat. In a small cup crumble the saffron into the milk and set aside for 3 hours. Prepare the rice as directed above. In a large pan that has a lid heat the butter or ghee over medium heat. Add the cardamom pods and cinnamon stick. Stir, then add the drained rice, stirring gently for about 3 minutes. Turn the heat down if the mixture gets too heavy. Add the water, saffron, turmeric, cloves, bay leaves, and raisins. Mix well. Cover with aluminum foil and the lid. Reduce the heat to very low and cook undisturbed for 25 minutes. Remove from the heat and allow the rice to rest for 10 minutes before serving. **Tip:** This rice is easy to make ahead and reheat.

Serves 4

Chilled Cucumber Soup

Great on hot summer evenings.

2	large cucumbers
8	to 9 tablespoons cold distilled water
2	tablespoons olive oil
1	tablespoon white wine vinegar
1	tablespoon minced fresh parsley
¾	teaspoon ground cumin
½	teaspoon dried thyme
	Chopped fresh mint for garnish

Peel the cucumbers. Cut them in half lengthwise and scrape out the seeds. Cut into 1-inch sections and purée (using a food processor is easiest), adding the water 1 tablespoon at a time. Transfer the purée to a bowl. In a small bowl mix the olive oil, vinegar, parsley, cumin, and thyme, then whisk into the purée. Refrigerate until well chilled. Garnish with fresh mint and serve cold.

Serves 4

Crab Quiche

4	farm fresh eggs
2	cups light cream
¼	teaspoon ground nutmeg
2	tablespoons unsalted butter
2	tablespoons minced scallions (green onions)
12	ounces crab meat (frozen is fine, just thaw and drain)
1	pastry crust

Preheat the oven to 425°F. In a large bowl combine the eggs, cream, and nutmeg, and beat with a wire whisk. Set aside. In a saucepan melt the butter over medium heat and add the minced scallions. Cook until tender. Blend into the egg mixture. Add the crab and mix well, and pour into the crust. Bake for 15 minutes, then reduce the oven temperature to 325°F and bake for another 35 minutes. Cool before serving.

Serves 6

Polish Barley Soup

1	cup pearl barley
2	quarts vegetable or chicken stock
¼	cup unsalted butter
2	carrots, sliced
1	stalk celery, chopped
1	pound button mushrooms, chopped
2	medium potatoes, chopped (skins on)
1	teaspoon parsley
	Fresh ground pepper to taste
1	cup sour cream (optional)

In a large saucepan combine the barley with 1 cup of the stock. Bring to a boil, then reduce the heat and simmer until all of the stock is absorbed and the barley is cooked. Add the butter and combine. In another pot cook the carrots, celery, mushrooms, and potatoes in the remaining stock. Do not boil. Add the barley and parsley and simmer for about 20 minutes. Add fresh ground pepper, and garnish with a dollop of sour cream, if desired. Serve.

Serves 4

Ayurvedic Curry

2   tablespoons olive oil or ghee

1   teaspoon whole mustard seed

1½ tablespoons curry (yellow type is best)

3   cloves garlic, finely chopped

1   ½-inch slice fresh ginger, minced

½   medium onion, finely chopped

1   teaspoon turmeric

1   14.5-ounce can organic crushed/chopped tomatoes

6   cups assorted raw or frozen vegetables, such as carrots, potatoes, green beans, peas, broccoli, cauliflower, eggplant, or squash

½   cup distilled water

In a large skillet heat the olive oil over medium heat. Add the mustard seed, curry, garlic, ginger, onion, and turmeric, and sauté until the seeds start to pop. Add the tomatoes and heat, stirring, until warm. Stir in the vegetables and water and simmer, covered, for approximately 15 minutes. Serve alone or on rice.

Serves 2

Cream of Tomato Soup

32 ounces tomatoes (fresh or canned—organic low- or no-sodium)

9 ounces vegetable or chicken broth

1 ounce unsalted butter

2 tablespoons raw organic sugar

1 tablespoon finely chopped onion

1 clove garlic, crushed

2 cups cream

Fresh ground pepper to taste

In a large pan combine the tomatoes, broth, butter, sugar, onion, and garlic. Simmer for 1 hour. In a double boiler heat the cream, then add to the hot tomato mixture. Blend well, add pepper, and serve.

Serves 4

6

Desserts

What would life be without sweets? Here are some safe bets that won't get in the way of your new healthy lifestyle. Enjoy!

Bread Pudding

4   to 5 slices Italian or French bread
1   large apple, cored, peeled, and
    thinly sliced
1   cup raisins, soaked in distilled
    water overnight, or until soft
1   cup pecan pieces

Sauce:
6   farm fresh egg yolks
¼   cup raw organic sugar
¼   cup raw organic honey
2   tablespoons unsalted butter
1   cup light cream

Preheat the oven to 350°F. In a 9-inch square glass baking dish combine the bread, apple slices, raisins, and pecans. Mix well, and set aside.

In the top of a double boiler (not over the heat yet) combine the egg yolks and sugar. Mix with a whisk until well blended. Add the honey and whisk together. Place the mixture over simmering water in the double boiler base. Cook, whisking constantly, for approximately 10 minutes, until the mixture is thoroughly warmed. Add the butter and cream and whisk constantly for another 5 to 8 minutes.

Remove from the heat and pour over the ingredients in the baking dish. Bake for 20 minutes, until golden brown. Cool. Serve as is, or pour some cream over each serving as an added delight.

Serves 4

Chocolate Madness

2	squares unsweetened organic chocolate, melted
½	cup organic flour
½	cup raw organic sugar
¼	cup unsalted butter, softened
1½	teaspoons real vanilla extract
¼	teaspoon baking powder
1	cup chopped walnuts
½	cup chopped pecans
½	cup chopped macadamia nuts
½	cup chocolate chips
½	cup white chocolate chips

Preheat the oven to 350°F. Line a baking sheet with a Silpat mat or use a nonstick baking sheet. In a large bowl mix together the melted chocolate, flour, sugar, butter, vanilla, and baking powder. Mix well. Add the walnuts, pecans, and macadamia nuts and mix well. Add the chips and mix well. Drop by teaspoonfuls about ½ inch apart on the prepared baking sheet. Bake for 10 minutes. Remove and set the cookies on wire racks to cool.

Makes 24 cookies

Baked Apples

4   medium apples of your choice
    Fresh ground cinnamon
    Raisins
    Chopped organic walnuts
4   tablespoons unsalted butter
    Light cream
    Fresh ground nutmeg

Preheat the oven to 350°F. Core the apples from the top, using a corer, but do not go all the way through. Place the apples in a glass baking dish with a little distilled water in the bottom. In the hole in the apples left by the core, sprinkle cinnamon, raisins, and walnuts, and top with 1 tablespoon of butter. Make sure your filling does not come over the top of the apple itself. Bake until golden and the apple is fork-tender. Remove from the oven and cool. Pour some cream over each apple and sprinkle with fresh ground nutmeg. Serve.

Serves 4

Honey Almond Pears

3 tablespoons sliced raw almonds

2 tablespoons raw organic honey

2 large ripe pears, halved lengthwise and cored, stem is optional

1 tablespoon unsalted butter

½ teaspoon vanilla powder

Light cream (optional)

Heat a large skillet over medium-high heat. Add the almonds and cook until lightly browned. Stir often to keep from scorching. Remove the almonds from the skillet and set them aside. Reduce the heat to medium and add the honey. Place the pears cut-side down on the honey and cook until fork-tender. Remove and place on 4 small dessert plates, cut-side up. Turn off the heat and add the butter and vanilla powder to the honey in the skillet. Heat through, then add the almonds. Stir. Spoon equal amounts of sauce over each pear and serve. If using cream, drizzle over each pear before serving.

Serves 4

Heather's Strawberry Pie

1 quart fresh-picked and ripe strawberries
3 tablespoons cornstarch
1 cup raw organic sugar
2 tablespoons fresh-squeezed lemon juice (one large lemon)
1 pre-cooked 9-inch pastry crust
Whipping cream (optional)

In a saucepan crush half of the strawberries, then stir in the cornstarch, sugar, and lemon juice. Cook over medium heat until the mixture is thickened and clear. Set aside to cool. Cut some of the remaining berries in half, saving the rest for the top of the pie. Fold the cut berries into the mixture. Pour into the pastry crust. Slice the remaining berries and arrange on the top of the pie. Chill fully before serving. Serve with a dollop of whipped cream, if desired.

Serves 6 (if you're willing to share)

Berry Cobbler

1 tablespoon unsalted butter

2 cups mixed berries (fresh is best but frozen will work)

1 cup flour

1 cup raw organic sugar

3 teaspoons baking powder

¼ cup oats

¾ cup 2 percent milk

Preheat the oven to 400°F. In an 8-inch square glass baking dish melt the butter. Spread the berries in the baking dish. In a bowl mix the flour, sugar, baking powder, oats, and milk. Pour the batter on top of the berries. Bake for 10 minutes, reduce the oven temperature to 300°F, and bake until golden.

Serves 4 to 6

Hawaiian Cake Pudding

1 loaf stale French bread, cubed

½ cup 2 percent milk

1 12-ounce can coconut milk (regular or lite)

4 farm fresh eggs, beaten

¼ cup macadamia nut halves

¼ cup shredded coconut

Preheat the oven to 350°F. In an 8-inch square glass baking dish spread the stale bread cubes. In a large bowl mix the milk, coconut milk, and eggs. Pour over the bread. Sprinkle the nut halves and shredded coconut on top, and bake until golden.

Serves 6

Honey Ice Cream

1   cup whole milk

2   cups organic heavy cream

4   egg yolks, beaten

½   cup raw organic honey (darker will give more flavor than light-colored honey)

1   cup chopped walnuts, pecans, or almonds

Fresh mint for garnish

In a saucepan combine the milk and cream over medium heat. Heat through. Slowly add the beaten egg yolks. Over low heat cook until the mixture is thick like a custard. Whisk in the honey. Strain and cool in the refrigerator for a minimum of 2 hours, preferably overnight. Pour the mixture into the canister of an ice cream maker and make the ice cream according to the manufacturer's directions. For harder ice cream put back into the freezer. Serve with a sprig of mint.

Serves 4

Summer Pudding

1 loaf sliced bread, crusts removed

Assorted berries, such as
blackberries, raspberries,
blueberries, or red currants

½ cup raw organic sugar

Whipped cream (optional)

Using a pudding basin (a dish that is deeper than it is wide), line the sides with slices of bread in a patchwork fashion until the sides are completely covered. In a saucepan boil the berries with the sugar until juicy and slightly mushy and aromatic. Pour the mixture into the bread-lined basin. Cover the top with more bread. Place a plate and a heavy object on top of the basin. Do not allow the pudding to ooze. Place in the refrigerator overnight. The next day the pudding should be one solid mass. Turn out onto a plate. Serve with whipped cream, if desired.

Serves 4

Heather's Incredible Triple-Berry Cheesecake

10 ounces frozen berry mix, thawed, or three kinds of fresh ripe berries, such as strawberries, blackberries, raspberries, or blueberries

1½ teaspoons cornstarch

Crust:

4 tablespoons unsalted butter, melted

1 cup organic graham cracker crumbs

3 tablespoons raw organic sugar

24 ounces cream cheese, softened (if not using organic, use only Philly)

¾ cup raw organic sugar

1 teaspoon vanilla powder

3 eggs

Sliced strawberries for garnish

Melted chocolate for garnish

Preheat the oven to 350°F. Using a stand mixer and attachment or a blender, purée the berries and cornstarch together. Heat over medium heat in a saucepan until thick; set aside to cool. To make the crust, in a small bowl combine the melted butter, graham cracker crumbs, and 3 tablespoons sugar. Press into the bottom of a 9-inch springform pan. Bake for 10 minutes. Cool.

Reduce the oven temperature to 300°F. In the mixer bowl with the paddle attachment combine the cream cheese, sugar, and vanilla powder until well blended. Add the eggs one at a time, mixing well before adding the next one. When the crust is fully cooled, add half of the cream cheese mixture to the base carefully. Make sure it is even and smooth. Add half of the cooled berry mixture in spoonfuls on top of the cheese. Add the remaining cheese batter on top of that, and finally the other half of the berry mixture. Twist a knife through the batter to create a swirl effect through the cheesecake. Bake for approximately 55 minutes. Allow to cool before serving. Best served the following day. Before serving arrange sliced strawberries on top and drizzle with melted chocolate.

Serves 6

Strawberry Bundles

16 ounces cream cheese, softened

6 ounces ripe strawberries, chopped

1 teaspoon lemon juice

¼ teaspoon vanilla powder

4 tablespoons raw organic sugar

¼ teaspoon ginger

Philo dough

Melted unsalted butter

Melted chocolate for garnish

In a mixing bowl combine the cream cheese, strawberries, lemon juice, vanilla powder, sugar, and ginger. Blend well and let sit for 30 minutes. Cut the frozen philo dough into 4-inch squares. Line the cups of a large nonstick muffin tin with the squares. Spoon some cream cheese mixture into the center of each square. Bring the corners of the dough together over the filling and press firmly with your fingers to close. Brush melted butter over the bundles and bake for 10 to 15 minutes, until golden and flaky. Drizzle with melted chocolate and serve warm or cool.

Serves 4

Mangos with Cream

1 to 2 ripe mangos
Cream
Raw organic honey

Peel the fruit and slice it into long slices lengthwise. Lay the slices on plates next to each other. Drizzle cream and honey over the fruit and serve. Simple and incredible.

Serves 2

African Bananas in Coconut Milk

4 bananas, peeled and sliced
1 teaspoon curry powder
½ teaspoon cinnamon
⅛ teaspoon ground cloves
1 to 1½ cups lite coconut milk

In a saucepan combine the bananas with the curry powder, cinnamon, and ground cloves. Pour in 1 cup of coconut milk and simmer over low heat until tender and the milk is absorbed. Add more coconut milk, if desired. Serve warm.

Serves 4

Irish Prune Cake

½ cup unsalted butter, softened
1 cup raw organic sugar
2 farm fresh eggs
2½ cups unbleached organic flour
¼ teaspoon nutmeg
1 teaspoon cinnamon
¼ teaspoon baking soda
3 teaspoons baking powder
1 cup 2 percent milk
1 cup cooked and chopped prunes

Preheat the oven to 350°F. In a large bowl blend together the butter and sugar. Add the eggs one at a time, blending well after each addition. In a separate bowl sift together the flour, spices, baking soda, and baking powder. Combine the mixtures, then add the milk. Blend well. Add the prunes and mix. Pour into a cake pan or glass baking dish and bake for approximately 30 minutes. Cool before serving.

Serves 4

American Indian Pudding

3   cups 2 percent organic milk
⅓   cup yellow cornmeal
¼   cup raw organic sugar
½   teaspoon cinnamon
½   cup raisins
1   tablespoon molasses
     Lite cream (optional)

Preheat the oven to 350°F. Butter an 8-inch square baking dish. In a saucepan heat the milk. In a bowl combine the cornmeal, sugar, and cinnamon. Add the milk and blend well. Mix in the raisins and molasses, and then pour into the prepared baking dish. Bake for just over 1 hour. Serve hot or cold. Pour cream on top for an extra treat.

Serves 4

7

Happy Holidays

Holiday time can be stressful. Add to that hepatitis C, and things can really get out of hand. Change that. Go for less stress, fewer parties, and less decadent food. The holidays can be happy, and taste good too!

Fall Harvest Muffins

1½ cups organic unbleached flour

1½ teaspoons baking powder

1 teaspoon baking soda

2 teaspoons ground cinnamon

1 teaspoon ground ginger

½ teaspoon ground nutmeg

⅛ teaspoon ground cloves

½ stick unsalted butter, softened

¾ cup raw organic honey

1 egg

1 cup pumpkin (cooked or organic canned, or use butternut squash for a smoother flavor)

1 cup walnuts or pecans

Preheat the oven to 325°F. Line a muffin tin with paper baking cups or use a nonstick muffin tin. In a medium bowl combine the flour, baking powder, baking soda, cinnamon, ginger, nutmeg, and cloves. Blend and set aside. In a large bowl beat the butter, honey, egg, and pumpkin until smooth. Add the dry mixture slowly, incorporating well. Add the nuts and mix. Spoon into the prepared muffin tin and bake for approximately 25 minutes or until a toothpick comes out clean. Place the muffins on a wire rack to cool before serving.

Makes 12

Butternut Soup

2 tablespoons unsalted butter
1 medium onion, chopped
2 garlic cloves, finely chopped
3 medium carrots, diced
2 celery stalks, diced
1 potato, peeled and diced
43 ounces chicken stock
1 medium to large butternut squash
Fresh ground pepper to taste

In a large stockpot melt the butter over medium heat. Add the onion and garlic, and cook until they release their aromas and the onion is clear. Add the carrots and celery, cooking and stirring until tender. Next add the potato, stock, and butternut squash. Blend well and bring to a boil. Simmer for approximately 40 minutes, until the veggies are soft. Remove from the heat and cool. Purée the mixture in a blender, reheat, and serve.

Serves 6

Cranberry Relish

¾ cup raw organic honey

½ cup raw organic sugar

3 cups fresh or frozen cranberries (thawed)

1 cup distilled water

½ cup peeled and chopped granny smith apple

Zest of 1 orange

Juice of 1 orange

½ cup chopped walnuts

½ cup raisins

In a medium pot add the honey, sugar, and cranberries to the water. Cook over medium heat until the berries begin to pop. Add the apple, zest, and juice, and cook for approximately 15 minutes, until everything is well blended and the berries are cooked down. Add the walnuts and raisins. Mix. Can be served warm or chilled.

Serves 8 to 10

Roasted Brussels Sprouts

2 pounds fresh Brussels sprouts
Olive oil
Fresh ground pepper to taste

Preheat the oven to 400°F. Line a baking sheet with a Silpat mat or lightly coat it with olive oil. Remove the exterior leaves from the Brussels sprouts. Place on the prepared baking sheet. Drizzle with olive oil and sprinkle with pepper. Roast for approximately 15 minutes, until the middles are fork-tender but the skins are browned and roasted nicely. **Tip:** Other vegetables, such as fennel, beets, or potatoes, can be prepared in the same way.

Serves 4

Amazing Stuffing

4	tablespoons unsalted butter
3	tablespoons olive oil
2	large onions, chopped
2	celery stalks, chopped
1	carrot, chopped
1	granny smith apple, chopped
2	tablespoons dried rosemary
1	tablespoon chopped fresh oregano
1	tablespoon chopped fresh sage
1	loaf stale French bread, cubed

In a large skillet over medium heat melt the butter. Add the olive oil, then sauté the onions, celery, carrot, and apple. When the onion turns clear and the other vegetables soften, add the rosemary, oregano, and sage. Sauté for a few minutes and add the bread. Mix well. Heat through. Remove, cool slightly, and stuff your turkey. Reserve the leftover stuffing to use as dressing; place it in a glass baking dish and cook in the oven next to the turkey until the top is browned. **Tip:** When the turkey is done, let it rest for 20 minutes before you try to carve it and remove the stuffing.

Fills a 12-pound bird, with some left to use as dressing

Autumn Mousse Pie

2	cups pumpkin, cut into small chunks and roasted (approximately 1 small pumpkin)
1	medium butternut squash, same as above
1	medium sweet potato, same as above
2	egg yolks
2	mashed bananas
1	cup heavy cream
1	cup raw organic sugar
½	teaspoon ground cinnamon
½	teaspoon ground nutmeg
½	teaspoon ground ginger
1	pastry crust, cooked and cooled

In the bowl of a stand mixer blend the pumpkin, squash, and sweet potato. In a small bowl combine about ½ cup of the pumpkin mixture with the egg yolks. Mix well, and add back into the rest of the pumpkin mixture. Add the mashed bananas, cream, sugar, cinnamon, nutmeg, and ginger. Blend well, but leave some texture. (If you prefer a smoother filling, purée the mixture.) Pour the filling into the pastry crust. Chill before serving.

Serves 6

Heather's Holiday Cheesecake

3   8-ounce packages cream cheese,
     softened
¾   cup raw organic sugar
1   teaspoon vanilla powder
3   eggs
1   teaspoon cinnamon
½   teaspoon nutmeg
1   9-inch graham cracker crust
     Crushed walnuts

Preheat the oven to 325°F. In the bowl of a stand mixer combine the cream cheese, sugar, and vanilla powder. Mix well. Add the eggs, one at a time. Add the cinnamon and nutmeg, and blend smooth. Line the crust with crushed walnuts. Pour the batter on top. Bake for 55 minutes. Cool and serve.

Serves 6

Honey Carrots

3	cups peeled and sliced carrots
2	tablespoons unsalted butter
¼	cup raw organic honey
2	teaspoons fresh chopped parsley

In a saucepan steam the carrots until tender, but not mushy. Place the carrots in a medium bowl and stir in the butter, honey, and parsley, mixing well. Serve.

Serves 4

Acorn Wedges

2 ripe acorn squashes
4 tablespoons unsalted butter
¼ cup organic maple syrup

Halve the squashes and remove the seed centers. Cut into
wedges. In a small saucepan melt the butter with the maple
syrup and heat until warm. Place the squash wedges in a baking
dish and pour the warmed syrup mixture on top. Refrigerate for
at least 1 hour, or overnight.

Preheat the oven to 400°F. Line a baking sheet with a Silpat
mat or lightly coat with butter. Place the squash wedges on the
baking sheet and roast until golden.

Serves 4

Holiday Scones

1¾ cups organic unbleached flour
1 tablespoon baking powder
1 cup oats
½ cup chopped pecans
½ teaspoon orange peel
8 tablespoons (1 stick) unsalted butter
¼ cup 2 percent milk
1 farm fresh egg
⅓ cup raw organic honey

Preheat the oven to 375°F. Line a baking sheet with a Silpat mat or lightly coat with butter. In a large bowl combine the flour and baking powder. Add the oats, pecans, and orange peel. Mix well. Cut the butter into 8 pieces, then cut into the dry mixture using two knives or a pastry blender, until coarse crumbs form. In a small bowl beat together the milk, egg, and honey with a whisk. Add to the dry ingredients, stirring with a fork until the dough begins to stick together. On a floured surface knead the dough 10 times. Flatten the dough into a circle approximately ¼ inch thick with your hand and cut into 8 wedges. Place the wedges on the prepared baking sheet and bake for 10 to 12 minutes. Serve warm.

Makes 8

Holiday Spinach

8   pounds fresh spinach, stems removed

¼   cup olive oil

1   cup pine nuts

⅔   cup dried currants, soaked in warm water for 30 minutes and drained on paper towels

     Fresh ground pepper to taste

In a large saucepan boil some water, then plunge the spinach, cooking for approximately 10 minutes. Drain and squeeze out the extra moisture. Allow to drain an additional 2 to 3 minutes. In a skillet heat the olive oil. Toss in the pine nuts. When they start to color add the currants and stir. Heat through. Add the spinach and mix. Heat well, season with pepper, and serve warm.

Serves 6

8

The World of Salads

Salad is a wonderful way to get various nutrients into one light meal. The ones you'll find here are good as side dishes, suppers, or even snacks. They also work well when entertaining non–hep C guests.

Chicken Salad

4 cups diced cooked chicken breast (boiled or baked)

1½ cups mayonnaise

1 teaspoon curry powder

1 tablespoon lemon juice

1 cup diced celery

1 cup green seedless grapes (whole or halved)

1 cup nuts (walnuts, almonds, hazelnuts)

In a large bowl combine all of the ingredients and blend well. Serve on a roll, in a scooped-out fresh tomato, or on a bed of salad greens.

Serves 4

Festival Salad

1	red bell pepper, chopped
1	yellow bell pepper, chopped
1	orange bell pepper, chopped
1	green bell pepper, chopped
3	scallions (green onions), sliced
1	avocado, peeled and sliced
¼	cup black olives
1	medium cucumber, sliced
1	tomato, chopped
½	cup garbanzo beans (chickpeas)
½	cup chopped parsley
	Salad dressing of your choice

In a large bowl toss all of the ingredients except the dressing together. Add any creamy low-sodium dressing of your choice. Coat well and serve.

Serves 4

Sweet Potato Salad

1 tablespoon olive oil

1½ pounds sweet potatoes, peeled and cut into chunks

⅓ cup chopped nuts (walnuts, almonds, pecans)

½ cup orange juice (fresh-squeezed is best)

1 teaspoon orange zest

⅓ cup golden raisins

3 tablespoons orange marmalade

1 granny smith apple, chopped (with skin)

2 tablespoons mayonnaise

Preheat the oven to 400°F. Drizzle the olive oil onto a baking sheet. Add the sweet potato chunks and toss to coat with the oil. Roast, turning as needed, until the potatoes start to brown. Place a Silpat mat on another baking sheet, spread out the nuts, and toast lightly, about 5 minutes. In a saucepan combine the orange juice, zest, and raisins. Over medium heat cook the mixture until the raisins are softened and the juice is reduced, about 10 minutes. Remove from the heat and stir in the marmalade. When the potatoes are ready, put in a large bowl, adding the apple and nuts. Mix well. Add the mayonnaise to the raisin mixture and stir. Pour over the potatoes and toss to coat. Serve warm or chill first.

Serves 6

Montana Winter Salad

3   cups broccoli florets
6   cups cauliflower florets
1   16-ounce package frozen organic peas
3   stalks celery, chopped
½   cup unsalted peanuts

Dressing:

1½ cups mayonnaise
¼   cup raw organic sugar
2   tablespoons lemon juice
½   cup Parmesan cheese (optional)

In a large bowl combine the broccoli, cauliflower, peas, celery, and peanuts. Toss. In a small bowl combine the mayonnaise, sugar, lemon juice, and Parmesan cheese (if desired). Mix well. Add to the salad bowl and toss to coat. Serve.

Serves 4

Cucumber Salad

1   cup organic sour cream

3   tablespoons finely chopped fresh chives

2   tablespoons fresh-squeezed lemon juice

3   large cucumbers, peeled and thinly sliced

Fresh ground pepper to taste

In a large bowl combine the sour cream, chives, and lemon juice. Blend well. Add the cucumber slices and incorporate into the mixture. Chill well. Add pepper just before serving.

Serves 6

Rice & Quinoa Salad

1 ¼ cups distilled water

½ cup organic wild rice, washed and drained

1 cup quinoa, washed (Quinoa is a grain from South America.)

2 carrots, grated

1 tablespoon fresh-squeezed lemon juice

3 tablespoons olive oil

¼ cup balsamic vinegar

2 cloves garlic, minced

2 tablespoons thinly sliced scallions (green onions)

1 tablespoon finely chopped fresh chives

¼ cup fresh parsley, chopped

Fresh ground pepper to taste

In a saucepan boil the water. Add the rice, cover, and simmer for 45 minutes. In a skillet over high heat dry roast the quinoa, moving it around with a wooden spoon until slightly browned and fragrant, about 5 minutes. In a bowl combine the grated carrots with the lemon juice and set aside. Increase the heat on the rice and bring it to a boil, add the quinoa, reduce to a simmer, and recover, cooking for 15 minutes.

In a bowl combine the olive oil, vinegar, garlic, scallions, and chives, and blend well. When the grains are cooked, allow to cool. Add the carrots and fluff with a fork. Put into a bowl and add the dressing, mixing well. Add the parsley and pepper. Serve warm or chilled.

Serves 6

California-Style Salad

2 teaspoons chopped parsley

½ head lettuce (not iceberg), shredded

½ head second kind of lettuce (not iceberg), shredded

2 large avocados, peeled and cut into chunks

¼ cup raisins

¼ cup apple, cored and chopped (not peeled)

1 cup Cheddar (or other) cheese cubes

Dressing:

¼ cup olive oil

Balsamic vinegar to taste

In a large salad bowl combine the parsley, lettuces, avocados, raisins, apple, and Cheddar cheese. Pour the olive oil into a glass measuring cup. Add the balsamic vinegar, and blend well with a fork. Pour over the salad. Allow the dressing to soak into the salad for 10 minutes before serving. **Variation:** You may want to add cubed or shredded grilled chicken to make this salad a meal.

Serves 8

Hawaiian Fruit Salad

¼ cup fresh-squeezed lime juice

¼ cup ginger syrup

4 medium papayas, peeled, seeded, and chopped

4 medium bananas, peeled and sliced

1 pineapple, peeled, cored, and chunked

¼ cup shredded coconut

Lite cream (optional)

In a large bowl combine the lime juice, ginger syrup, papayas, bananas, pineapple, and coconut. Blend well. Chill and serve with cream, if desired.

Serves 8

Mozzarella Tomato Salad

6   medium organic ripe tomatoes,
    sliced or chunked

6   medium-sized mozzarella balls in
    water, drained, and sliced

1½ cups shredded radicchio and
    romaine lettuce

Dressing:

2   tablespoons olive oil

2   tablespoons balsamic vinegar

1   teaspoon ground oregano

1   teaspoon ground basil

Fresh basil for garnish (optional)

In a large bowl combine the tomatoes, mozzarella, and lettuce.
In a small bowl mix the olive oil, balsamic vinegar, oregano,
and basil. Pour over the salad. Garnish with fresh basil leaves
and serve.

Serves 6

Pasta Salad

1	pound pasta, any kind
1	tomato, diced
1	orange or yellow bell pepper, diced
1	cucumber, diced
½	cup sliced scallions (green onion)
1	12-ounce container mozzarella balls, sliced
1	tablespoon chopped fresh basil
1	tablespoon chopped fresh parsley
	Low fat, low-sodium Italian dressing

Cook the pasta according to package directions. Drain and cool. In a large bowl combine the pasta, tomato, bell pepper, cucumber, scallions, mozzarella cheese, basil, and parsley. Toss to blend. Add dressing and chill before serving.

Serves 6

Grape Salad

½ cup sour cream
¼ cup raw organic sugar
1 teaspoon vanilla powder
1 large bunch purple or blue
    seedless grapes, washed and
    dried

In a large bowl combine the sour cream, sugar, and vanilla powder. Let sit for 10 minutes. Fold in the grapes and serve.

Serves 4

Red Beet Salad

1 tablespoon vinegar
½ teaspoon raw organic honey
4 medium beets, cooked and diced
1 small onion, finely chopped
1 scallion (green onion), sliced

In a large bowl combine the vinegar and honey. Add the beets, onion, and scallion. Mix well. Chill and serve cold.

Serves 4

Potato Salad

3   pounds potatoes, cooked and drained
1   cup diced celery
3   tablespoons cider vinegar
4   farm fresh eggs, boiled and chopped

Dressing:

1   pint organic sour cream
1   tablespoon vinegar
2   teaspoons raw organic sugar
½   teaspoon pepper
3   teaspoons Dijon mustard
1   small onion, chopped
1   clove garlic, minced

In a large bowl combine the potatoes, celery, cider vinegar, and eggs, blending well. In a second bowl make the dressing: combine the sour cream, vinegar, sugar, pepper, mustard, onion, and garlic. Mix well. Pour the dressing over the potato mixture. Chill before serving.

Serves 6

Frisée Salad

1 granny smith apple, cored and chopped

1 large orange, peeled and divided into sections or cut into chunks

1 head of frisée (also called endive) lettuce, separated

3 scallions (green onions), sliced

2 tablespoons cider vinegar

¼ cup olive oil

In a large bowl combine all of the ingredients. Let stand for 15 minutes, then serve.

Serves 6

Rice Salad

3 tablespoons olive oil
1 large onion, sliced
3 cloves garlic, chopped
1 cinnamon stick
1 bay leaf
2 cardamom pods
4 cloves
½ teaspoon garam masala
3½ cups boiling distilled water
½ cup raisins
2 cups basmati rice, rinsed 5 times, soaked for 30 minutes, and drained for 30 minutes
½ pound fresh raw green beans, ends and strings removed

In a large skillet heat the olive oil over medium heat. Add the onion and garlic, and cook until soft. Add the cinnamon, bay leaf, cardamom, cloves, and garam masala, and cook until blended. Add the rice, then add the water and raisins. Allow the water to boil, stir, and cover the pot with aluminum foil, then the lid. Cook for 15 minutes. Remove from the heat and allow the mixture to settle, covered, for 10 minutes—do not open the lid. Using a fork, fluff the rice into a bowl. Add the green beans, blend, and allow to come to room temperature. Serve.

Serves 4

Spinach Salad

1 cup dried figs, quartered, no stems
 Distilled water
¼ cup diced shallots
1½ cups olive oil
4 cups baby spinach
¼ pound blue cheese, crumbled or chunked

In a small pot over medium heat rehydrate the figs in distilled water. Allow to cool, then cut into small pieces. In a medium bowl combine the figs, shallots, and olive oil. Toss in the baby spinach and blue cheese. Serve.

Serves 2

9

Extras

This chapter is full of all the goodies that just didn't fit anywhere else.

Cucumber Cups

1 cup yogurt
1 14- to 16-inch cucumber, peeled
3 scallions (green onions), minced
⅓ cup minced fresh dill
¼ pound thinly sliced smoked
   salmon

In a fine sieve set over a bowl drain the yogurt. Place the strained yogurt in a small bowl and cover tightly with plastic wrap to prevent a skin from forming. Allow to sit overnight.

Slice the peeled cucumber into 16 ¾-inch slices, and with a melon baller scoop out the centers to create cups. Allow to drain on paper towels for 10 minutes. In a bowl combine the drained yogurt, scallions, and dill. Pat the cucumber cups dry and fill with the yogurt mixture. Cut the salmon into ½-inch strips. Roll the strips up and place on top of the cups. Can be made in advance and chilled before serving.

Makes 16

Strawberry Surprise

1   10-ounce package organic frozen strawberries
2   tablespoons lemon juice
¼   cup raw organic sugar
1   cup organic sour cream

In a large freezer-proof bowl combine the strawberries, lemon juice, sugar, and sour cream. Freeze for 2 hours, stirring twice.
Variation: You can also use this recipe with raspberries, black-berries, or blueberries.

Serves 4

Norman Flat Bread

This is an adaptation of a recipe that my mother used to make as a special treat for springtime entertaining. It was a favorite of both her children and her guests, and usually was gone long before the night was over.

2	cups organic unbleached flour
2	farm fresh eggs, beaten
16	tablespoons unsalted butter, cut into pieces and softened
1	cup light cream
1	tablespoon rosemary tips
¼	cup pine nuts (pignoli)
1	egg yolk, beaten

Preheat the oven to 425°F. Line a baking sheet with a Silpat mat or lightly coat with butter. Place the flour in a large bowl. Make a well in the center of the flour and add the eggs, then the butter and cream. Blend. Stir in the rosemary and pine nuts. Knead well with your fingers until a smooth dough forms. Cover and let the dough stand for 30 minutes. Roll out the dough on a floured surface and fold into quarters. Roll again and repeat the folding. Shape the dough into a ball, cover, and let rest for 15 minutes. Roll into a circle, about 10 inches wide. Score a cross lightly in the top and lay on the prepared baking sheet. Brush the round with the beaten egg yolk and bake for 30 minutes or until browned. Cool slightly before serving.

Serves 8

Hot Cider

1 gallon high-quality organic cider
2 orange peels fresh from the
orange
Juice from the same 2 oranges
4 cinnamon sticks
8 cloves
Bit of powdered ginger, or chunk
of fresh

In a large pot combine all of the ingredients. Simmer over medium heat until warmed through. Serve warm.

Makes 1 gallon

Quick Appetizer

1   loaf of bread (stale works best)
     Olive oil
1   red apple, sliced
1   basket of fresh figs, halved
     Brie, Gorgonzola, and Pepper
     Jack cheese

Using a cookie cutter (can use different shapes for fun), cut out the centers of each slice of bread. Drizzle olive oil on the bread. Place a slice of apple or fig on the cutout, then a slice of cheese. Make various combinations. Broil in the oven until the cheese melts and the bread is toasted, about 8 minutes.

Serves 4 to 6

Pretzels

1 ⅓ cups plus 2 tablespoons warm water

1   package dry yeast

⅓   cup brown sugar

5   cups organic flour

½   cup baking soda

Preheat the oven to 475°F. Butter 2 baking sheets. In a large mixing bowl mix 2 tablespoons water with the yeast. Allow to sit for a moment. Add the remaining water and the brown sugar. Blend. Gradually add the flour, stirring to blend until a ball forms. Turn out onto a floured work surface and knead until smooth. In a saucepan bring 2 quarts of water and the baking soda to a boil. Cut the dough into 20 small pieces, then roll them into logs about ½-inch thick. To make the pretzel create a U shape, then cross the ends, twisting at the middle. Fold the ends back to meet the U and press the dough securely. Drop into the boiling water for about 30 seconds, remove and place on the buttered cookie sheet. When all are cooked and on the sheets, bake in the oven for 8 to 10 minutes. Make sure they are golden before removing. Serve warm or cool.

Makes 20

Corn Bread

1   cup organic flour

1   cup organic yellow fine or coarse cornmeal

3   tablespoons raw organic sugar

1½   teaspoons baking powder

1   tablespoon paprika

1   large egg, lightly beaten

1   cup 2 percent milk

¼   cup olive oil

½   medium onion, chopped

Preheat the oven to 400°F. Coat a baking dish with unsalted butter. In a large bowl combine the flour, cornmeal, sugar, baking powder, and paprika, and set aside. In a small bowl combine the beaten egg, milk, olive oil, and chopped onion. Pour the wet ingredients into the dry and blend. Spread the batter into the prepared baking dish and bake for 25 minutes or until a toothpick comes out clean and the edges are slightly browned. Serve warm—with chili!

Serves 8

Bean & Cheese Quesadillas

2 medium-sized flour tortillas

1 14.5-ounce can organic refried beans (low salt)

1½ cups Cheddar or Pepper Jack cheese

½ medium onion, chopped

½ medium tomato, chopped

Sour cream

Preheat the oven to 400°F. Line a baking sheet with a Silpat mat or lightly coat it with olive oil. Lay 1 tortilla flat and layer ingredients on top. Start with the beans, then add the cheese, onion, and tomato. Finish with a dollop of sour cream and top with the second tortilla. Place on the prepared baking sheet. Cook for about 15 minutes, until the cheese is fully melted and the top is crisp. Cool slightly. Cut with a pizza wheel and serve.

Serves 2

Quick Onion Tarts

12 thin slices of bread, crusts removed
2 tablespoons unsalted butter
1 tablespoon extra-virgin olive oil
2 large onions, thinly sliced
1 pound Gruyère cheese, shredded (can substitute Swiss cheese)
Fresh ground pepper to taste

Preheat the oven to 350°F. Line a baking sheet with a Silpat mat or lightly coat with olive oil. Place the bread slices on the baking sheet. Bake for a few minutes, until toasted. Remove and set aside. In a skillet melt the butter and olive oil. Add the onions and cook until caramelized, about 15 to 20 minutes (add water if you want a saucy caramel). Turn on the broiler. Place the onions on top of the toasted bread. Cover with Gruyère cheese and add pepper. Broil until the cheese bubbles. Serve warm.

Serves 4

Pizza Dough

1 cup distilled water (110°F)
1 ¼-ounce envelope active dry yeast
1 teaspoon raw organic sugar
2 tablespoons extra-virgin olive oil
3 cups unbleached high-gluten flour

In a large bowl combine the water, yeast, sugar, and 1 tablespoon olive oil. Set aside and allow the mixture to foam. Add half of the flour to the mixture and mix by hand until blended. The mixture should be smooth. Add the remaining flour slowly, blending by hand until all the flour is used and the dough is smooth and slightly sticky. Turn the dough out onto a floured surface. Knead by hand, making sure the dough stays smooth and just a little sticky. Coat a clean bowl with 1 tablespoon olive oil. Place the dough ball in the bowl and cover. Set aside until the dough doubles, about 1 hour and 30 minutes. Ready to use.

Makes one large pizza, 6 Stromboli, or 2 calzones

Calzones

	Olive oil
2	tablespoons unsalted butter
2	large sweet onions, sliced
1	red bell pepper, sliced
1	green or other color bell pepper, sliced
1	small package button mushrooms, cleaned and sliced
3	tablespoons minced garlic (fresh is best)
1	teaspoon dried Italian oregano
1	teaspoon dried basil
1	teaspoon dried Italian parsley
	Pizza dough (see recipe, p. 129)
½	cup sliced black olives
2	cups grated Provolone cheese
2	cups grated mozzarella cheese
2	cups ricotta cheese
1	large farm fresh egg, beaten and mixed with 1 tablespoon water
	Grated Parmesan cheese

Preheat the oven to 375°F. Line a baking sheet with a Silpat mat or lightly coat with olive oil. In a large skillet over medium heat drizzle some olive oil and add 1 tablespoon butter. When the butter is melted, add the onions and bell peppers. When the vegetables are wilted, add the remaining 1 tablespoon butter and the mushrooms. Sauté until golden. Add the garlic and herbs. Blend well and heat through. Remove from the heat and set aside.

At this point your dough should have doubled in size. Punch it down. Place it on a floured surface and divide in half. Roll out one half of the dough in a rectangular shape. Spread one-half of the onion mixture on the dough, leaving a 1-inch border all the way around. Top with half of the black olives, and half of the three cheeses. Dip a pastry brush in the egg mixture and brush the edge all the way around the dough. Fold the dough over and pinch together the edges to seal. Use a fork to press the edges. Brush the top with the egg wash and place on the prepared baking sheet. Repeat the process with the second half of the dough and ingredients and set it beside the first calzone. Allow both to rise, about 30 minutes. Bake for about 30 minutes, until the dough is golden. Remove and allow to rest for 10 minutes before cutting and serving.

Serves 6

Mushroom and Spinach Roulade

Olive oil

1 tablespoon unsalted butter

10 ounces organic frozen chopped spinach

1 pound fresh spinach

4 farm fresh eggs, separated

Fresh ground pepper to taste (optional)

¼ cup grated Parmesan cheese

For filling:

1 tablespoon unsalted butter

1½ cups button mushrooms, sliced

1 tablespoon unbleached flour

⅔ cup 2 percent milk

¼ teaspoon nutmeg

Fresh ground pepper to taste

Preheat the oven to 400°F. Line a jelly roll pan or a bread pan (12 x 8-inch is best) with parchment paper. Lightly coat the parchment with olive oil. In a skillet heat 1 tablespoon butter and cook the spinach until softened. Drain and place in a large bowl. Add the egg yolks, beating into the spinach. Add pepper, if desired. In a bowl whisk the egg whites until they just begin to hold their shape. Fold into the spinach mixture. Sprinkle some Parmesan cheese into the prepared pan, then add the spinach mixture. Sprinkle the remaining Parmesan on top. Cook for about 10 minutes.

Now prepare the filling. In a small skillet heat 1 tablespoon butter. Add the mushrooms and cook until soft. Add the flour, stirring to blend. Slowly add in the milk and stir until the sauce thickens. Add the nutmeg and pepper. Remove the spinach from the oven and invert onto a sheet of waxed paper. Spread the mushroom filling over the spinach and gently roll it up. Cut into thick slices and serve warm.

Serves 4

Cucumber Relish

1	large cucumber, peeled, seeded, and chopped
4	fresh ripe plum (Roma) tomatoes, chopped
2	cloves garlic, minced
¼	cup organic Italian chopped fresh parsley
1	teaspoon chopped fresh marjoram
1	teaspoon chopped fresh thyme
2	tablespoons fresh-squeezed lemon juice
	Fresh ground pepper to taste

In a large bowl combine all of the ingredients. Blend well. Cover and refrigerate until cold. Serve.

Serves 4

Garlic Butter

1   cup unsalted butter, softened

3   cloves garlic, pressed

¼   teaspoon chopped fresh Italian oregano

½   teaspoon chopped fresh Italian parsley

In a small bowl combine all of the ingredients. Blend well. Cover or put in a mold, and refrigerate until firm. Delicious on any bread.

Serves 8

Honey Butter

1 cup unsalted butter, softened
½ cup raw organic honey

In a small bowl combine the butter and honey. Blend well. Serve soft. This spread is best on dark breads.

Serves 8

Guacamole

2   large ripe organic avocados,
    mashed
3   tablespoons fresh-squeezed lime
    juice
1   tablespoon chopped fresh cilantro
3   tablespoons chopped scallions
    (green onions)
3   tablespoons mayonnaise

In a bowl combine all of the ingredients and blend well. Cover
and chill before serving. This recipe easily doubles.

Serves 4

Pineapple Milkshakes

3 cups organic French vanilla ice cream
10 ounces fresh pineapple chunks
½ cup organic 2 percent milk
Sprig of fresh mint for garnish

In a blender combine the ice cream, pineapple, and milk. Blend. Pour into frosty glasses, top with mint, and serve.

Serves 2

Mushroom Sauce

3   tablespoons unsalted butter
1   teaspoon lemon juice
½   cup button mushrooms (or any
    other type), cleaned and sliced
¼   cup unbleached flour
1¼ cups 2 percent milk
    Fresh ground pepper to taste

In a skillet combine 1 tablespoon butter and the lemon juice.
Blend, add the mushrooms, and sauté. In a small saucepan melt
the remaining butter, stir in the flour, and cook for 1 minute,
stirring constantly. Remove from the heat and stir in the milk
and pepper. Return to the heat and bring to boil for 2 minutes,
still stirring. Remove from the heat and add the mushrooms.
Pour over food, or serve on the side.

Serves 2

Steamed Corn on the Cob

Corn loses its flavor quickly after being picked. To ensure the best flavor do not allow corn to sit out. Buy corn that has been picked within 24 hours and use it right away. If you are unable to use right away, store in airtight plastic bags in the refrigerator, but no more than 2 days, or you will lose the flavor.

1	tablespoon olive oil
1	tablespoon Asian sesame oil
2	cloves garlic, crushed
1	teaspoon chili flakes (optional)
1	teaspoon pepper
2	tablespoons chopped fresh cilantro
1	tablespoon onion powder
4	fresh ears corn, husks removed

In a large bowl combine the olive oil, sesame oil, garlic, chili flakes (if desired), pepper, cilantro, and onion powder. Allow the corn to sit in the mixture overnight, turning once in a while to coat each side.

Wrap each corn cob in parchment paper and twist the ends. Cook in a covered steamer over rapidly simmering water until cooked, about 8 minutes. Remove and serve warm.

Serves 4

Old-Fashioned American Apple Butter

4	pounds tart apples
2	cups cider
4	cups (approximately) raw organic sugar
2	teaspoons cinnamon
1	teaspoon ground cloves
1	teaspoon ground ginger
½	teaspoon ground allspice

Cut the apples into quarters. *Do not peel or seed.* In a stainless pot combine the apples with the cider and bring to a boil over high heat. Reduce the heat to low and cover the pot. Simmer the apples, stirring occasionally, for 25 minutes or until soft. Remove from the heat and mash the apples through a sieve. Measure the pulp and transfer to a heavy saucepan. Add ½ cup sugar for every cup of pulp. Now add the cinnamon, cloves, ginger, and allspice. Cook over medium heat, stirring occasionally, for about 4 hours. **Test:** 1 tablespoon of the butter sticks to a saucer when inverted. Ladle into sterilized jars. Cool at room temperature. Place in the refrigerator for use, or seal the top with paraffin wax, then cover tightly and store in cool dry place. Will last for several months.

Makes 3 pints

Herbed Mayonnaise

2   tablespoons cider vinegar

1   egg yolk

1   whole egg, hard-boiled

2   cups French-style mustard

2   tablespoons finely chopped fresh basil leaves

2   tablespoons finely chopped fresh oregano

1   tablespoon finely chopped fresh Italian parsley

   Fresh ground pepper to taste

1   teaspoon raw organic sugar

   Extra-virgin olive oil

¼   cup plain organic yogurt

In a blender or food processor combine the cider vinegar, egg yolk, hard-boiled egg, and mustard, and process for 10 seconds. Add the chopped herbs, pepper, and sugar, and process for another 5 seconds. Leaving the blender on, add the olive oil slowly to produce a smooth but thick sauce. Add more olive oil to adjust the thickness to your personal taste. Leave the blender running while slowly adding the yogurt. Process for several seconds after the yogurt has been added. Spoon into a jar with an acid-proof lid and refrigerate overnight before using.

Serves 4

appendix

Shopping Resources

Here are some places to look for items that are all-natural or "organically produced." Local farmers markets, farms, and health food stores (listed in your phone book) are also good places to look. I have also included some places to get seeds if you want to grow your own herbs or vegetables.

united states

Bass Lake Cheese Factory (Wisconsin)
(800) 368-2437
www.blcheese.com

Maharishi Ayur-Ved Products International
(800) 255-8332
www.mapi.com

Wheat Montana
(800) 535-2798
www.wheatmontana.com

G.B. Russo & Son (Michigan)
(800) 767-8776
www.gbrusso.com

Pasta Cheese Gourmet Food Shop
(800) 386-9198
www.pastacheese.com

Grace's Marketplace (New York City)
(212) 737-0600
www.gracesmarketplace.com

Horizon Herbs (Oregon)
(541) 846-6704
www.horizonherbs.com

Hardbody Nutrition
(800) 378-6787
www.hardbodynutrition.com

Shop Natural Store (Arizona)
www.shopnatural.com

Country Sun Natural Foods
(California)
(650) 324-9190
www.countrysun.com

Flowers by the Sea (California)
(707) 877-1722
www.fbts.com

Morningside Farms (Tennessee)
(615) 563-2353
www.morningsidefarm.com

Door to Door Organics
(Pennsylvania)
(888) 283-4443 (2VEGGIE)
www.doortodoororganics.com

Diamond Organics (Colorado)
(888) 674-2642
www.diamondorganics.com

Kalyx Herbs, Foods, Supplements,
Bath, & Aromatherapy (New York)
www.kalyx.com

Green Barley (Nevada)
(866) 463-1844
www.greenbarley.com

canada

Green Earth Organics (Toronto)
www.greenearthorganics.com

united kingdom

www.freshfood.co.uk

www.organic-connections.co.uk

united states farmers markets and farms

www.localharvest.org

Dekalb Farmer's Market (Georgia)
(404) 377-6400

Barry Farm
(419) 228-4640
www.barryfarm.com

Renaissance Acres Organic Herb
Farm (Michigan)
(734) 449-8336
www.provide.net/~raohf/

index

W

About the Author

Heather Jeanne has twelve years of experience in the restaurant field. Her recipes have been published in numerous magazines, and she has won local prizes and awards for her great-tasting, creative foods. The founder of her own business, she lives in Laurel, Montana, where she cares for her father, who was diagnosed with late-stage hepatitis C more than six years ago.